CENTERS for MEDICARE & MEDICAID SERVICES

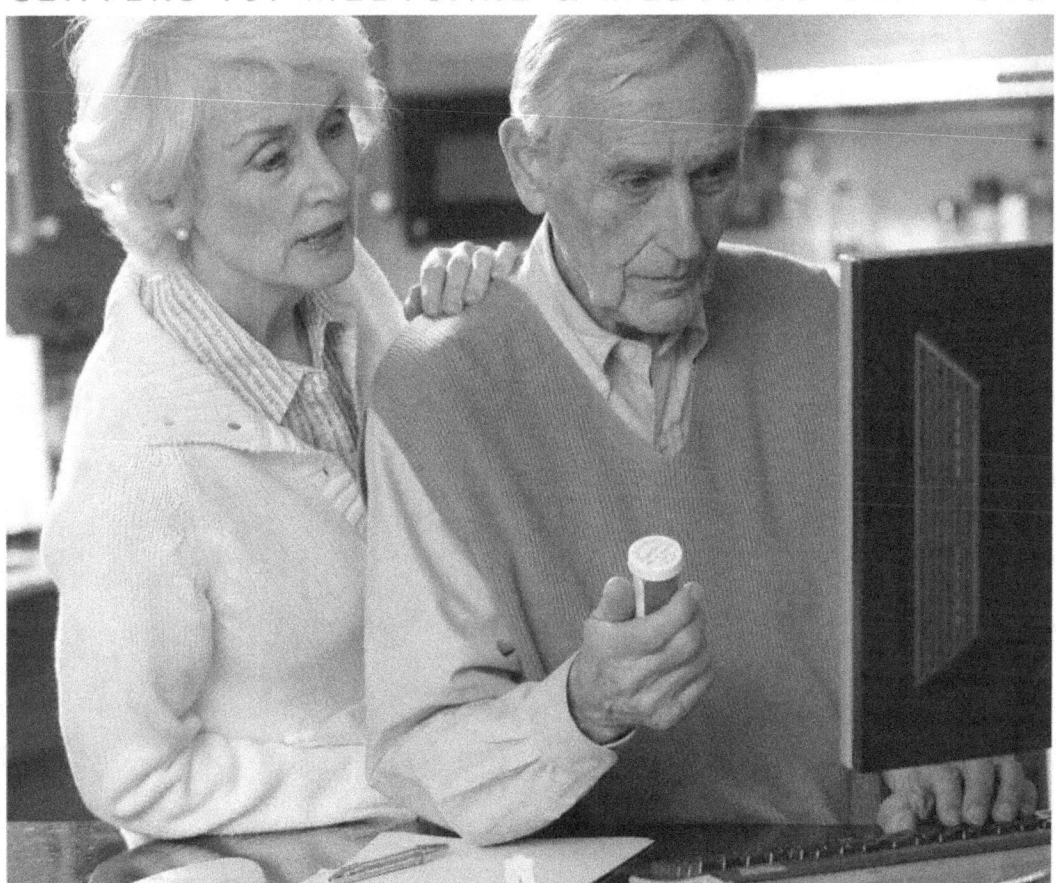

Your Guide to Medicare
Prescription Drug Coverage

This official government booklet tells you:

- How your coverage works

- How to get Extra Help if you have limited income and resources

- How Medicare drug coverage works with other drug coverage you may have

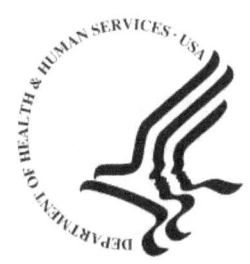

Table of Contents

Table of Contents (continued)

Section 5: 3 Steps to Choosing a Medicare Drug Plan . . 67

Section 6: Tips for Using Your New Medicare Drug Coverage 71

Table of Contents (continued)

The Basics

Medicare prescription drug coverage adds to your Medicare health care coverage

Medicare prescription drug coverage (Part D) helps you pay for both brand-name and generic drugs. Medicare drug plans are offered by insurance companies and other private companies approved by Medicare.

You can get coverage 2 ways:

1. Medicare Prescription Drug Plans (sometimes called "PDPs") add prescription drug coverage to Original Medicare, some Medicare Private Fee-for-Service (PFFS) Plans, some Medicare Cost Plans, and Medicare Medical Savings Account (MSA) Plans.

Words in red are defined on pages 83–86.

2. Some Medicare Advantage Plans (like HMOs or PPOs) or other Medicare health plans offer prescription drug coverage. You generally get all of your Medicare Part A (Hospital Insurance), Medicare Part B (Medical Insurance), and Part D through these plans. Medicare Advantage Plans that offer prescription drug coverage are sometimes called "MA-PDs."

In this booklet, the term "Medicare drug plans" means all plans that provide Medicare prescription drug coverage.

The Basics

Medicare prescription drug coverage adds to your Medicare health care coverage (continued)

Joining a drug plan

To join a Medicare Prescription Drug Plan, you must have Medicare Part A (Hospital Insurance) **or** Medicare Part B (Medical Insurance). To join a Medicare Advantage Plan or other Medicare health plan with prescription drug coverage, you must have Part A **and** Part B. You must also live in the service area of the Medicare health plan or drug plan you want to join.

All Medicare drug plans must give at least a standard level of coverage set by Medicare. However, plans offer different combinations of coverage and cost sharing. Medicare drug plans may differ in the prescription drugs they cover, how much you have to pay, and which pharmacies you can use.

Words in red are defined on pages 83–86.

If you decide to join a Medicare drug plan, compare plans in your area and choose one that meets your needs. If you don't join a Medicare drug plan when you're first eligible for Medicare, and you don't have drug coverage that's expected to pay, on average, at least as much as standard Medicare prescription drug coverage (called creditable prescription drug coverage), you may have to pay a late enrollment penalty if you join later. The penalty is in addition to your premium each month for as long as you have a Medicare drug plan.

The Basics

Pick the drug coverage that meets your needs

Everyone with Medicare has to make a decision about prescription drug coverage. If you don't use a lot of prescription drugs now, you still may want to think about joining a Medicare drug plan to help lower your drug costs now and help protect against higher costs in the future. If you're new to Medicare and already have other drug coverage, you have new options to think about. If you aren't new to Medicare, you may

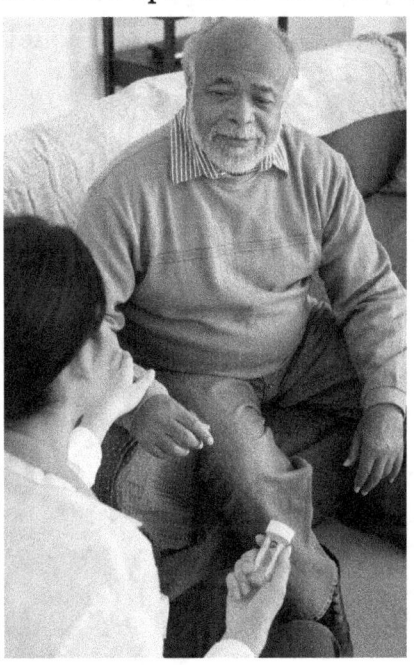

want to look at your options to find drug coverage that meets your needs. You can join or switch Medicare drug plans between October 15–December 7 each year, with your coverage beginning January 1 of the following year.

Consider all your drug coverage choices before you make a decision. Look at the drug coverage you may already have, like coverage from an employer or union, TRICARE, the Department of Veterans Affairs (VA), the Indian Health Service, or a Medicare Supplement Insurance (Medigap) policy. Compare your current coverage to Medicare drug coverage. The drug coverage you already have may change because of Medicare drug coverage, so consider all your coverage options.

If you have (or are eligible for) other types of drug coverage, read all the materials you get from your insurer or plan provider. Talk to your benefits administrator, insurer, or plan provider before you make any changes to your current coverage.

Note: Drug coverage is insurance. Doctor samples, discount cards, free clinics, or drug discount websites **aren't** drug coverage.

For details about how Medicare drug coverage may affect other coverage, see Section 4.

The Basics

Get help with your choices

- Visit the Medicare Plan Finder at Medicare.gov/find-a-plan to find plans in your area that cover your drugs and pharmacies that can fill your prescriptions.

- Call your State Health Insurance Assistance Program (SHIP) for free personalized health insurance counseling. To get the most up-to-date SHIP phone numbers, visit shiptacenter.org or call 1-800-MEDICARE (1-800-633-4227). TTY users should call 1-877-486-2048.

- Call 1-800-MEDICARE.

Words in red are defined on pages 83–86.

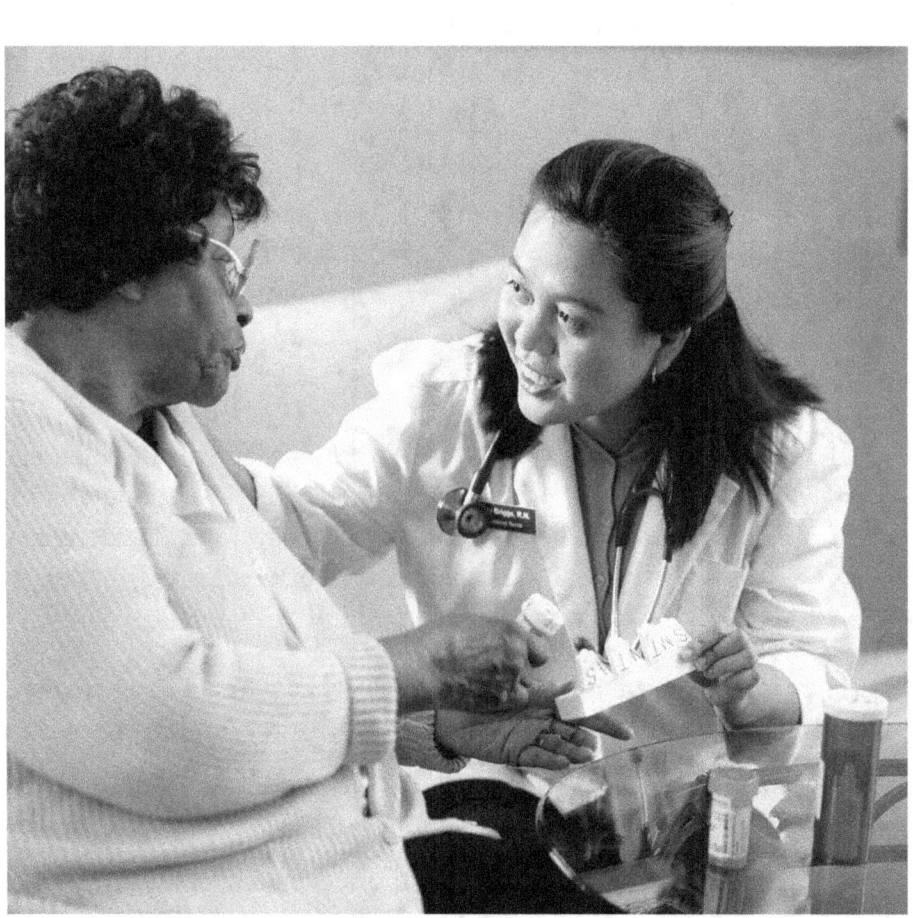

How Medicare Drug Coverage Works

Compare these things to find a plan that meets your needs:

Coverage

Medicare drug plans cover generic and brand-name drugs. All plans must cover the same categories of drugs, but generally plans can choose which specific drugs are covered in each drug category.

Cost

Plans have different monthly premiums. How much you pay for each drug depends on which plan you choose. If you have limited income and resources, you may qualify for Extra Help from Medicare with paying your drug plan costs. For more information on Extra Help, see Section 3.

Convenience

Check with the plan to make sure the pharmacies in the plan are convenient to you. Many plans also allow you to get your drugs by mail. If you spend part of the year in another state, see if the plan will cover you there.

Quality

Use the Medicare Plan Finder at Medicare.gov/find-a-plan to get plan ratings in different categories, like customer service. You can also call 1-800-MEDICARE (1-800-633-4227) for plan rating information. TTY users should call 1-877-486-2048.

2 How Medicare Drug Coverage Works

How is Part D coverage different from Part B coverage for certain drugs?

Medicare Part B (Medical Insurance) includes limited drug coverage. It doesn't cover most drugs you get at the pharmacy. You'll need to join a prescription drug plan to get Medicare coverage for drugs for most chronic conditions, like high blood pressure.

Part B covers certain drugs, like injections you get in a doctor's office, certain oral cancer drugs, and drugs used with some types of durable medical equipment—like a nebulizer or external infusion pump. Under very limited circumstances, Part B covers certain drugs you get in a hospital outpatient setting. You pay 20% of the Medicare-approved amount for these covered drugs. Part B also covers the flu and pneumococcal shots. Generally, Medicare drug plans cover other vaccines, like the shingles vaccine, needed to prevent illness.

Note: Generally, self-administered drugs you get in an outpatient setting (like in an emergency room, observation unit, surgery center, or pain clinic) aren't covered by Medicare Part A (Hospital Insurance) or Part B. Your Medicare drug plan may cover these drugs under certain circumstances. You'll likely need to pay out-of-pocket for the entire cost of these drugs and send in a claim to your drug plan for a refund. Call your plan for more information. Also, visit Medicare.gov for more information on how Medicare covers self-administered drugs you get in a hospital outpatient setting.

What plans are available in my area?

Get information about specific drug plans in your area by visiting Medicare.gov/find-a-plan or by calling 1-800-MEDICARE (1-800-633-4227). TTY users should call 1-877-486-2048. For more information on how to compare plans and join one that meets your needs, see Section 5.

How Medicare Drug Coverage Works

How much will my drug coverage cost?

Medicare drug plans have different coverage and costs, but all must offer at least a standard level of coverage set by Medicare. How much you actually pay for Medicare drug coverage depends on which drugs you use, which Medicare drug plan you join, whether you go to a pharmacy in your plan's network, and whether you get Extra Help paying for your drug costs. Contact the plan(s) you're interested in to get specific cost information.

Your drug coverage costs are affected by:

Words in red are defined on pages 83–86.

- Monthly premium
- Yearly deductible
- Copayments or coinsurance
- Coverage gap (also called the "donut hole")
- Catastrophic coverage

Monthly premium

Most drug plans charge a monthly fee that differs from plan to plan. You pay this fee in addition to the Part B premium. If you belong to a Medicare Advantage Plan (like an HMO or PPO) or a Medicare Cost Plan that includes Medicare drug coverage, the monthly premium may include an amount for drug coverage.

Some people with Medicare may pay a higher monthly premium based on their income. If you reported a modified adjusted gross income of more than $85,000 (individuals and married individuals filing separately) or $170,000 (married individuals filing jointly) on your 2014 IRS tax return (the most recent tax return information provided to Social Security by the IRS), you'll have to pay an extra amount for your Medicare drug coverage, called the income-related monthly adjustment amount (IRMAA). You'll pay this extra amount in addition to your monthly Part D plan premium.

Social Security will send you a letter if you have to pay for this extra amount. Check the chart on the next page for the amount you'll have to pay each month.

How Medicare Drug Coverage Works

If your yearly income in 2014 was

File individual tax return	File joint tax return	File married & separate tax return	You pay each month (in 2016)
$85,000 or less	$170,000 or less	$85,000 or less	Your plan premium
above $85,000 up to $107,000	above $170,000 up to $214,000	N/A	$12.70 + your plan premium
above $107,000 up to $160,000	above $214,000 up to $320,000	N/A	$32.80 + your plan premium
above $160,000 up to $214,000	above $320,000 up to $428,000	above $85,000 up to $129,000	$52.80 + your plan premium
above $214,000	above $428,000	above $129,000	$72.90 + your plan premium

Your adjustment amount will get taken out of your monthly Social Security, Railroad Retirement, or Office of Personnel Management check, no matter how you usually pay your plan premium. If that amount is more than what's in your check, you'll get a bill from Medicare each month.

If you don't pay your entire Part D premium (and the extra amount), you may be disenrolled from your Part D plan. You must pay both the extra amount and your plan's premium each month to keep Medicare drug coverage.

If you have to pay a higher amount for your Part D premium and you disagree, visit socialsecurity.gov, or call 1-800-772-1213. TTY users should call 1-800-325-0778.

Yearly deductible

The deductible is what you pay for your drugs before your plan begins to pay. No Medicare drug plan may have a deductible more than $360 in 2016. Some plans charge no deductible.

How Medicare Drug Coverage Works

You pay copayments or coinsurance for your drugs after you pay the deductible. You pay your share, and your plan pays its share for covered drugs.

Usually, the amount you pay for a covered drug is for a one-month supply of a drug. However, you can request less than a one-month supply for most types of drugs. You might do this if you're trying a new medication that's known to have significant side effects or you want to get the refills for all your drugs on the same refill schedule. If you do this, the amount you pay is reduced based on the quantity you actually get. Talk with your prescriber to get a drug for less than a one-month supply.

Words in red are defined on pages 83–86.

Coverage gap (also called the "donut hole")

The Affordable Care Act has made Medicare drug coverage more reasonably priced with the gradual closing of the coverage gap. You reach the coverage gap after you and your plan have spent a certain amount of money for covered drugs. When you're in the coverage gap, you may pay more costs for your drugs out-of-pocket, up to a limit. **Not everyone will reach the coverage gap.** Your yearly deductible, coinsurance or copayments, and what you pay in the coverage gap all count toward this out-of-pocket limit. The limit doesn't include the drug plan's premium or what you pay for drugs that aren't on your plan's formulary (drug list).

You won't need to pay all out-of-pocket costs when you're in the coverage gap. In 2016, your plan will cover at least 5% of the cost of covered brand-name drugs, and the drug manufacturer will give a 50% discount, for a combined savings of at least 55% on these brand-name drugs. The amount you pay and the 50% discount you get from the manufacturer both count as out-of-pocket spending that will help you get out of the coverage gap.

The coverage gap will continue to shrink each year until 2020, when you'll only pay 25% for both covered generic and brand-name drugs when in the gap.

How Medicare Drug Coverage Works

For each month that you fill a prescription, your drug plan mails you an "Explanation of Benefits" (EOB) notice, which tells you how much you've spent on covered drugs and if you've reached the coverage gap. In 2016, your EOB notice will also show the 55% discount on covered brand-name drugs you buy in the coverage gap.

Catastrophic coverage

The amount you pay for drugs and the 50% discount in the coverage gap both count toward your out-of-pocket limit. Once you reach your plan's out-of-pocket limit, you come out of the coverage gap and you automatically get "catastrophic coverage." Under catastrophic coverage, you only pay a small coinsurance amount or a copayment for the rest of the year.

The example below shows the costs for covered drugs in 2016 for a plan that has a coverage gap:

Ms. Smith joined the ABC Prescription Drug Plan. Her coverage began on January 1, 2016. She doesn't get Extra Help and uses her Medicare drug plan membership card when she buys drugs.

Monthly premium—Ms. Smith pays a monthly premium throughout the year.			
1. Yearly deductible	**2. Copayment or coinsurance**	**3. Coverage gap**	**4. Catastrophic coverage**
Ms. Smith pays the first $360 of her drug costs before her plan starts to pay its share.	Ms. Smith pays a copayment, and her plan pays its share for each covered drug until their **combined** amount (plus the deductible) reaches $3,310.	Once Ms. Smith and her plan have spent $3,310 for covered drugs, she's in the coverage gap. In 2016, she gets a 55% discount on covered brand-name prescription drugs that counts as out-of-pocket spending, and helps her get out of the coverage gap. For 2016, she also gets an additional 5% coverage from her plan on covered brand-name drugs and 42% coverage on covered generic drugs while in the coverage gap.	Once Ms. Smith has spent $4,850 out-of-pocket for the year, her coverage gap ends. Now, she only pays a small copayment or coinsurance for each drug until the end of the year.
→	→	→	→

2 How Medicare Drug Coverage Works

Visit the Medicare Plan Finder at Medicare.gov/find-a-plan to view estimated yearly costs for each plan and your costs per drug for each month.

How can I pay my plan premium?

You can pay your premium by:

- Signing up to have it deducted from your checking or savings account.

- Charging it to a credit or debit card.

- Having your plan bill you each month directly. Some plans bill in advance for next month's coverage. Send your payment to the plan—not to Medicare. Contact your plan for their payment address.

Words in red are defined on pages 83–86.

- Having funds withheld from your Social Security payment. Contact your plan—not Social Security—to ask for this payment option. It may take up to 3 months to start, and it's likely the first 3 months of premiums will be collected at one time.

  - If you get Extra Help to pay part of your drug plan premium, Social Security may withhold your share of the monthly premiums.

  - **Note:** If you're in an employer health plan and your plan pays part of your drug plan premium, Social Security can't withhold your share of the monthly premiums.

> **Example of Social Security withholding:** Ms. Brown's monthly drug plan premium is $25, and her coverage begins in January. Her first premium payment of $75 is collected in March. It includes her premium for January, February, and March. After March, only one month of premium payments ($25) will be withheld from her Social Security payment each month.

If you qualify for Extra Help, some or all of your drug plan premiums may be covered. For more information, see Section 3.

How Medicare Drug Coverage Works

When can I join, switch, or drop a drug plan?

You can join, switch, or drop a Medicare drug plan:

- **During your 7-month Initial Enrollment Period, when you first become eligible for Medicare.** You can join a Medicare drug plan during the 7-month period that begins 3 months before you turn 65, includes the month you turn 65, and ends 3 months after the month you turn 65. Your coverage will begin the first day of the month after you ask to join a plan. If you join during one of the 3 months before you turn 65, your coverage will begin the first day of the month you turn 65.

- **During the 7-month period around your 25th month of disability.** If you get Medicare due to a disability, you can join a Medicare drug plan during the 7-month period that begins with your 22nd month of disability and ends with your 28th month of disability. Your coverage will begin the first day of the month after you ask to join a plan. You'll have another chance to join when you turn 65 (see above).

- **During Open Enrollment, between October 15–December 7 each year.** Your coverage begins January 1 the following year, as long as the plan gets your request during Open Enrollment.

- **At any time if you qualify for Extra Help.** This includes people who have Medicare and Medicaid, belong to a Medicare Savings Program, get Supplemental Security Income (SSI) benefits, and those who apply and qualify. Your coverage will begin the first day of the month after you qualify for Extra Help and ask to join a plan.

Note: In certain limited circumstances, you may be able to join, drop, or switch to another Medicare drug plan at other times. For example, you may be able to switch at other times if:

- You permanently move out of your drug plan's service area.
- You lose creditable prescription drug coverage.
- You enter, live in, or leave a nursing home.
- You want to switch to a plan with a 5-star overall quality rating. Quality ratings are available on Medicare.gov.
- Medicare considers your plan a "poor performer" (got a star rating under 3 stars for 3 or more years in a row).

How Medicare Drug Coverage Works

If you currently have Medicare drug coverage, you may want to review your coverage each fall. If you're happy with your coverage, cost, and customer service, and your Medicare drug plan is still offered in your area, you don't have to do anything to continue your coverage for another year. However, if you decide another plan will better meet your needs, you can switch to a different plan.

How do I switch plans?

All you need to do is join a new plan. You **don't** need to tell your current drug plan you're leaving or send them anything because joining a different Medicare drug plan, at the times listed on the previous page, disenrolls you from your current drug plan. Your new Medicare drug plan should send you a letter telling you when your coverage with your new plan begins.

How do I join a plan?

Contact the company that offers the plan. You may be able to enroll on the plan's website, or by mailing or faxing a completed enrollment form to the plan.

You can also enroll directly by visiting Medicare.gov/find-a-plan/questions/enroll-now.aspx, or by calling 1-800-MEDICARE (1-800-633-4227). TTY users should call 1-877-486-2048. Visit Medicare.gov/find-a-plan, or call 1-800-MEDICARE to get a list of Medicare plans in your area.

To join a Medicare drug plan, you'll need to give your Medicare number and the date your Medicare Part A (Hospital Insurance) and/or Medicare Part B (Medical Insurance) coverage started, which you'll find on your Medicare card.

Note: Medicare drug plans aren't allowed to call you to enroll you in a plan. Call 1-800-MEDICARE to report a plan that does this.

Words in red are defined on pages 83–86.

What's the Part D late enrollment penalty?

The late enrollment penalty is an amount that's added to your Part D premium if, at any time after your Part D initial enrollment period is over, there's a period of 63 or more days in a row when you don't have Part D or other creditable prescription drug coverage.

Note: If you get Extra Help, you don't pay a late enrollment penalty.

How Medicare Drug Coverage Works

How much is the late enrollment penalty?

Words in
red are
defined
on pages
83–86.

Currently, the late enrollment penalty is calculated by multiplying the 1% penalty rate times the "national base beneficiary premium" ($34.10 in 2016) times the number of full, uncovered months you were eligible to join a Medicare drug plan but didn't and went without other creditable prescription drug coverage.

The final amount is rounded to the nearest $.10 and added to your monthly premium. The "national base beneficiary premium" may go up each year, so the penalty amount may also go up each year. In addition to your premium each month, you may have to pay this penalty for as long as you have a Medicare drug plan.

Example:

Mrs. Martinez didn't join a drug plan when she was first eligible—by May 2013. She doesn't have prescription drug coverage from any other source. She joined a Medicare drug plan during the 2015 Open Enrollment Period, and her coverage began on January 1, 2016.

Since Mrs. Martinez was without creditable prescription drug coverage from July 2013–December 2015, her penalty in 2016 is 31% (1% for each of the 31 months) of $34.10 (the national base beneficiary premium for 2016), which is $10.57. The monthly penalty is rounded to the nearest $.10, so she'll be charged $10.60 each month in addition to her plan's monthly premium in 2016.

Here's the math:

.31 (31% penalty) × $34.10 (2016 base beneficiary premium) = $10.57

$10.57 (rounded to the nearest $0.10) = $10.60

$10.60 = Mrs. Martinez's monthly late enrollment penalty for 2016

When you join a Medicare drug plan, the plan will tell you if you owe a penalty and what your premium will be.

How do I avoid paying a penalty?

- **Join a Medicare drug plan when you're first eligible,** or have other creditable prescription drug coverage at that time.

- **Don't go 63 days or more in a row without a Medicare drug plan or other creditable prescription drug coverage.** Creditable prescription drug coverage could include drug coverage from a former employer or union, TRICARE, the Department of Veteran Affairs (VA), or the Indian Health Service. Your plan must tell you each year if your drug coverage is creditable. It may send you this information in a letter, or let you know in a newsletter or other piece of mail. Keep this information, because you may need it if you join a Medicare drug plan later.

- **Tell your Medicare drug plan when you join if you have other creditable prescription drug coverage.** When you join a Medicare drug plan, the plan may send you a letter asking if you have creditable prescription drug coverage if the plan believes you went 63 or more days in a row without other creditable prescription drug coverage. Complete the form and return it by the deadline in the letter. If you don't tell your plan about your creditable prescription drug coverage, you may have to pay a penalty.

Is my prescription drug coverage through the Marketplace considered creditable health insurance?

The Health Insurance Marketplace helps uninsured people find health coverage, and the Small Business Health Options Program (SHOP) Marketplace helps businesses provide health coverage to their employees.

Prescription drug coverage in a Marketplace or SHOP Marketplace plan isn't required to be creditable prescription drug coverage. However, all private insurers offering prescription drug coverage, including Marketplace and SHOP plans, are required to determine if their prescription drug coverage is creditable each year and let you know in writing.

For more information on the Marketplace or SHOP Marketplace, visit HealthCare.gov.

2 How Medicare Drug Coverage Works

What information do I need to join a Medicare drug plan?

- Name, birth date, and permanent home address
- Information found on your Medicare card (like your Medicare number)
- How you want to pay your plan premiums
- Other insurance information and any creditable coverage notices

You may be asked for this information when you join a Medicare drug plan, but it's optional and not required to process your enrollment:

- Email address
- Name and information for an emergency contact
- Name, address, and phone number of nursing home or institution where you live (if applicable)

Once you join a plan, the company will send you specific materials you'll need, like a membership card, member handbook, formulary (drug list), pharmacy provider directory, and complaint and appeal procedures.

Will I get a separate card for my Medicare drug plan?

Words in red are defined on pages 83–86.

When you join a Medicare Prescription Drug Plan that works with Original Medicare, the plan will mail you a separate card to use when you fill your prescriptions. You'll still use your Medicare card for hospital and doctor services. If you join a Medicare Advantage Plan (like an HMO or PPO) or other Medicare health plan with drug coverage, you'll also get a new card to use when filling your prescriptions and for hospital and doctor visits.

What if I need to fill a prescription before I get my membership card?

Within 2 weeks after your plan gets your completed application, you'll get a letter letting you know it got your information. Within 5 weeks, you should get a welcome package with your membership card. If you need to go to the pharmacy before your membership card arrives, you can use any of these as proof of membership:

- The acknowledgement, confirmation, or welcome letter you got from the plan
- An enrollment confirmation number you got from the plan, and the plan name and phone number
- A temporary card you may be able to print from MyMedicare.gov

Also bring your Medicare and/or Medicaid card and a photo ID, like your driver's license. If you qualify for Extra Help, see page 43 for more information about what you can use as proof of Extra Help. If you don't have any of the items above, and your pharmacist can't get your drug plan information any other way, you may have to pay out-of-pocket for the entire cost of your drugs. **Save the receipts and contact your plan if you do pay for your drugs out-of-pocket— you may be able to get back some of the cost or have the amount credited toward your out-of-pocket costs.**

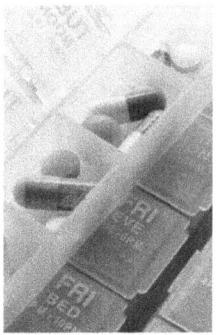

Once you choose a plan, enroll early in the month. This gives the Medicare drug plan time to mail you important information, like your membership card, before your coverage becomes effective. This way, even if you go to the pharmacy on your first day of coverage, you can fill your prescriptions without delay.

How Medicare Drug Coverage Works

Where can I fill my prescriptions?

Each company that offers a Medicare drug plan has a list of pharmacies you can use. If you want to continue filling prescriptions at the same pharmacy you use now, check to see if the pharmacy is on the plan's list. You can visit Medicare.gov, or call the plan, your pharmacy, or 1-800-MEDICARE (1-800-633-4227) to see if your pharmacy works with the plan you want to join. TTY users should call 1-877-486-2048.

Once you join a Medicare drug plan, the company will send you a pharmacy provider directory. Generally, you must go to one of these pharmacies for your plan to cover your drugs. Medicare requires plans to have network pharmacies for you to choose from. Plans can't make you use a mail-order pharmacy, but you may have this option and want to use it. You may find using a mail-order pharmacy to be a cost effective and convenient way to fill prescriptions for drugs you take every day.

Can I use an automatic refill mail-order service to get my drugs?

Some people with Medicare get their drugs by using an "automatic refill" service that automatically delivers prescription drugs when you're about to run out.

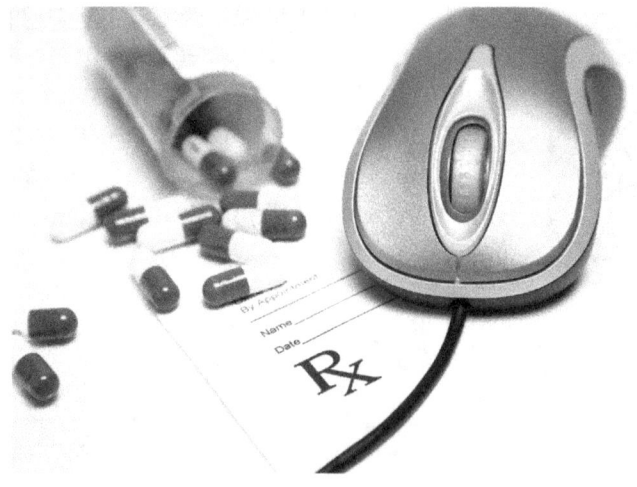

How Medicare Drug Coverage Works

Plans will get your approval to deliver a prescription drug (new or refill) unless you ask for the refill or request the new prescription. Some plans may ask you for your approval every year so that they can send you your drugs without asking you before each delivery. Other plans may ask you before every delivery.

This policy doesn't affect refill reminder programs where you go in person to pick up the drug, and it doesn't apply to long-term care pharmacies that give out and deliver prescription drugs.

Note: Be sure to give your pharmacy the best way to reach you, so you don't miss the refill confirmation call or other communication.

Contact your plan if you get any unwanted prescription drugs through an automated delivery program. You may be eligible for a refund for the amount you were charged. Call 1-800-MEDICARE (1-800-633-4227) if you experience any problems using automatic delivery and billing. TTY users should call 1-877-486-2048.

What are the special rules for people with End-Stage Renal Disease (ESRD)?

If you have End-Stage Renal Disease (ESRD) and you're in Original Medicare, you can join a Medicare Prescription Drug Plan. You generally can't join a Medicare Advantage Plan (like an HMO or PPO) except:

- If you're already in a Medicare Advantage Plan when you develop ESRD. You can stay in it or join another plan offered by the same company under certain circumstances.
- If you're a member of a health plan (like through a former employer or union) offered by the same company that offers one or more Medicare Advantage Plans. You may be able to join one of their Medicare Advantage Plans when you develop ESRD.
- If you've had a successful kidney transplant. You may be able to join a Medicare Advantage Plan.

How Medicare Drug Coverage Works

Words in red are defined on pages 83–86.

If you have End-Stage Renal Disease (ESRD) and are in a Medicare Advantage Plan (like an HMO or PPO), and the plan leaves Medicare or no longer provides coverage in your area, you have a one-time right to join another Medicare Advantage Plan, but you don't have to use this right immediately. If you go directly to Original Medicare after your plan leaves or stops providing coverage, you may use this right later as long as the plan accepts new members.

Also, you may be able to join a Medicare Special Needs Plan (SNP), a type of Medicare Advantage Plan for people with certain chronic diseases and conditions or who have specialized needs, if one is available in your area.

If you have ESRD and join a Medicare Prescription Drug Plan, Medicare Part B (Medical Insurance) will pay for some of the drugs you need, like injectable drugs and their oral forms, and biologicals including erythropoiesis-stimulating agents used for dialysis. Part D will continue to cover most ESRD-related drugs that are available only in oral form.

Visit Medicare.gov for more information if you have ESRD. You can also call 1-800-MEDICARE (1-800-633-4227). TTY users should call 1-877-486-2048.

What drugs are covered by Medicare drug plans?

Each plan may cover different drugs, so there's no single formulary (drug list) that fits all plans. All Medicare drug plans must make sure the people in their plan can get medically necessary drugs to treat their conditions. Drug lists, prior authorization, step therapy, and quantity limits are some of the coverage rules plans use to make sure certain drugs are used correctly and only when medically necessary. These coverage rules are described below and on the following pages.

Drug lists

Most Medicare drug plans have their own list of covered drugs, called a formulary. Plans cover both generic and brand-name drugs. Although Medicare drug plans aren't required to cover certain drugs, like drugs used for weight loss, weight gain, or erectile dysfunction, some plans may cover them as an added benefit. Also, drug plans generally don't pay for over-the-counter drugs. However, some states may cover over-the-counter drugs if you have Medicaid.

How Medicare Drug Coverage Works

To make sure people with different medical conditions can get the drugs they need, drug lists for each plan must include a range of drugs in each prescribed category. All Medicare drug plans generally must cover at least 2 drugs per drug category, but the plans can choose which specific drugs they cover. Plans are required to cover almost all drugs within these protected classes: antipsychotics, antidepressants, anticonvulsants, immunosuppressants, cancer drugs, and HIV/AIDS drugs.

A Medicare drug plan can make some changes to its drug list during the year if it follows guidelines set by Medicare. Your plan may change its drug list during the year because drug therapies change, new drugs are released, and new medical information becomes available.

Note: A plan isn't required to tell you in advance if it removes a drug from its drug list because the Food and Drug Administration (FDA) is taking the drug off the market for safety reasons, but it'll let you know afterward.

If the change involves a drug you're currently taking, your plan must do one of these:

- Provide written notice to you at least 60 days prior to the date the change becomes effective.
- At the time you request a refill, provide written notice of the change and a 60-day supply of the drug under the same plan rules as before the change.

You may need to change the drug you use or pay more for it. In some cases, you can keep taking the drug until the end of the year. You can also ask for an exception. See page 77.

Note: Since early 2016, in most cases, your prescribers need to be enrolled in Medicare or have an "opt-out" request on file with Medicare for your drugs to be covered by your Medicare drug plan. If your prescriber isn't enrolled or has "opted-out," you'll still be able to get a 3-month temporary fill of your prescription. This will give your prescriber time to enroll, or you time to find a new prescriber who's enrolled. Contact your plan or your prescribers for more information.

2 How Medicare Drug Coverage Works

If you use a drug not on your plan's drug list, you'll have to pay full price instead of a copayment or coinsurance unless you qualify for a formulary exception. All Medicare drug plans have negotiated to get lower prices for the drugs on their drug lists, so using those drugs will generally save you money. Also, using generics instead of brand-name drugs may save you money.

Generic drugs

The FDA says generic drugs are copies of brand-name drugs and are the same as those brand-name drugs in dosage form, safety, strength, route of administration, quality, performance characteristics, and intended use. Generic drugs use the same active ingredients as brand-name drugs. Generic drug makers must prove to the FDA that their product performs the same way as the corresponding brand-name drug. In some cases, there may not be a generic drug the same as the brand-name drug you take, but there may be a generic drug that will work as well for you. Talk to your doctor or other prescriber (a health care provider who's legally allowed to write prescriptions).

Tiers

To lower costs, many plans place drugs into different "tiers" on their formularies (drug lists). Each tier costs a different amount. A drug in a lower tier will cost you less than a drug in a higher tier. Each plan can divide its tiers in different ways.

Example:

- Tier 1–Generic drugs. Tier 1 drugs cost the least.
- Tier 2–Preferred brand-name drugs. Tier 2 drugs cost more than Tier 1 drugs.
- Tier 3–Non-preferred brand-name drugs. Tier 3 drugs cost the most.

Your plan's drug list might not include a drug you take. However, in most cases, you can get a similar drug that's just as effective.

Words in red are defined on pages 83–86.

Prior authorization

You may need drugs that require prior authorization. This means before the plan will cover a particular drug, your doctor or other prescriber must first show the plan it's medically necessary for you to have that particular drug. Plans also do this to be sure these drugs are used correctly. Contact your plan about its prior authorization requirements, and talk with your prescriber.

Step therapy

Step therapy is a type of coverage rule. In most cases, you must first try a certain less-expensive drug on the plan's formulary (drug list) that's been proven effective for most people with your condition before you can move up a "step" to a more expensive drug. For instance, some plans may require you first try a generic drug (if available), then a less expensive brand-name drug on their drug list before you can get a similar, more expensive, brand-name drug covered.

However, if your prescriber believes that because of your medical condition it's medically necessary for you to be on a more expensive step therapy drug without trying the less expensive drug first, you or your prescriber can contact the plan to request an exception. Your prescriber must give a statement supporting the request. If the request is approved, the plan will cover the more expensive drug.

Example:

> **Step 1**–Dr. Smith wants to prescribe an ACE inhibitor to treat Mr. Mason's heart failure. There's more than one type of ACE inhibitor. Some of the drugs Dr. Smith considers prescribing are brand-name drugs covered by Mr. Mason's Medicare drug plan. The plan rules require Mr. Mason to use a generic drug, lisinopril, first. For most people, the generic drug works as well as the brand-name drugs.

> **Step 2**–If Mr. Mason takes lisinopril but has side effects or limited improvement, Dr. Smith can provide that information to the plan to request approval to cover a brand-name drug that Dr. Smith wants to prescribe. If approved, Mr. Mason's Medicare drug plan will then cover the requested brand-name drug.

Quantity limits

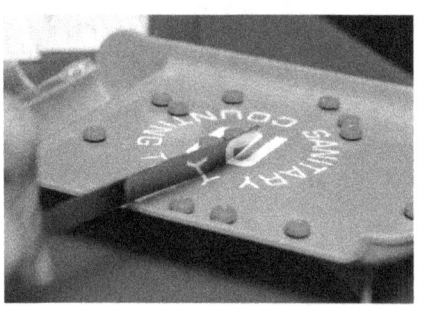

For safety and cost reasons, plans may limit the amount of drugs they cover over a certain period of time. For example, most people prescribed heartburn medication take 1 tablet per day for 4 weeks. Therefore, a plan may cover only an initial 30-day supply of heartburn medication. Should you need more tablets, you may need your doctor or other prescriber's help in providing information for a refill.

If your prescriber believes that, because of your medical condition, a quantity limit isn't medically appropriate, you or your prescriber can contact the plan to ask for an exception. If the plan approves your request, the quantity limit won't apply to your drug for the rest of the plan year.

What if I'm taking a drug that isn't on my plan's drug list when my drug plan coverage begins?

Generally, your drug plan will give you a one-time, temporary supply of your current drug during your first 90 days in a plan. Plans must give you this temporary supply so that you and your prescriber have time to find another drug on the plan's formulary (drug list) that will work as well as what you're taking now, or you or your prescriber can contact the plan to ask for an exception. There may be different rules for people who move into or already live in an institution (like a nursing home or long-term care hospital).

However, if you already tried similar drugs on your plan's drug list and they didn't work, or if your prescriber decides you need a certain drug because of your medical condition, you or your prescriber can contact your plan to ask for an exception as soon as your coverage begins. Also, you or your prescriber can ask for an exception if your prescriber thinks you need to have a coverage rule, like a quantity limit waived. If the plan agrees to your request, it'll cover the drug. If your plan doesn't agree to the exception, you can appeal the plan's decision. For more information on appeals, see pages 74–80.

2 How Medicare Drug Coverage Works

What if I join a plan, and then my doctor changes my prescription?

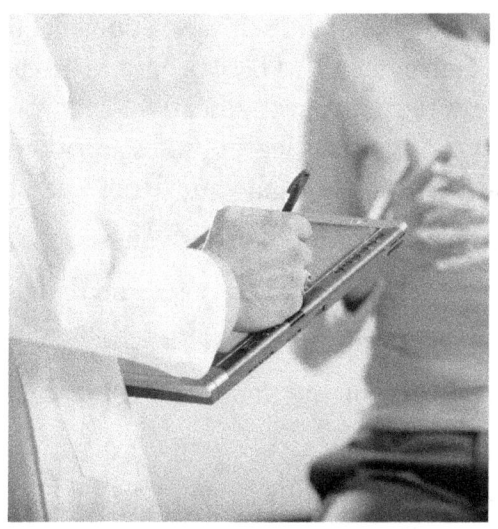

Your doctor or other prescriber may need to change your prescription or prescribe a new drug. If your doctor prescribes electronically, he or she can check which drugs your drug plan covers through his or her electronic prescribing system. If your doctor doesn't prescribe electronically, give him or her a copy of your Medicare drug plan's current formularies (drug lists).

Words in red are defined on pages 83–86.

If your doctor needs to prescribe a drug not on your Medicare drug plan's drug list and you don't have any other health coverage that covers outpatient prescription drugs, you or your doctor can ask the plan for an exception. For more information on exceptions, see page 77.

If your plan still won't cover a specific drug you need, you can file an appeal. If you want to get the drug before your appeal is decided, you may have to pay out-of-pocket for the entire cost of the drug. Keep the receipt and give a copy of it to the person deciding your appeal. If you win the appeal, the plan will pay you back. For more information about what to do if a plan won't cover a drug you need, see page 76–77.

Plans can change their drug list and costs for drugs. Call your plan or look on your plan's website to find the most up-to-date Medicare drug list and costs.

If I take medications for different medical conditions, am I eligible for Medication Therapy Management?

If you're in a Medicare drug plan and take medications for different medical conditions, you may be eligible to get services, at no cost to you, through a Medication Therapy Management (MTM) program. This program helps you and your doctor make sure that your medications are working to improve your health. A pharmacist or other health professional will give you a comprehensive medication review of all your drugs and talk with you about:

- How to get the most benefit from the drugs you take.
- Any concerns you have, like medication costs and drug reactions.
- How best to take your medications.
- Any questions or problems you have about your prescription drug and over-the-counter medication.

You'll get a written summary of this discussion to have available when you talk with your health care providers. The summary has a medication action plan that recommends what you can do to make the best use of your medications, with space for you to take notes or write down any follow-up questions. You'll also get a personal medication list that will include all of the medications you're taking and why you take them.

Your drug plan may enroll you in this program if you meet all of these conditions:

1. You have multiple chronic health conditions.
2. You take several different medications.
3. Your medications have a combined cost of more than $3,507 per year. This dollar amount (which can change each year) is estimated based on your out-of-pocket costs and the costs your plan pays for the medications each calendar year. Your plan can help you find out if you may reach this dollar limit.

Visit Medicare.gov/find-a-plan to get general information about program eligibility for your Medicare drug plan or for other plans that interest you. Contact each drug plan for specific details.

How to Get Extra Help

Ways to qualify for Extra Help

The chart on the following page shows different ways you may qualify for Extra Help, depending on your situation. It includes many, but not all, of the types of letters that Medicare sends, by color and name.

If you get one or more of these letters, keep them in case you need to show them to your plan as proof that you qualify for Extra Help.

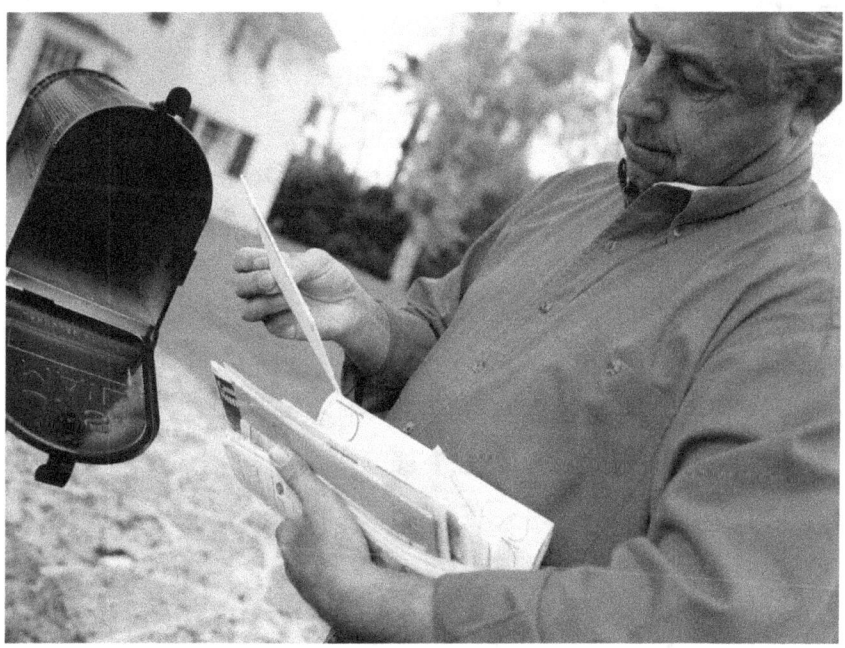

3 How to Get Extra Help

When you	Medicare will mail you a letter that's this color	Official name
Automatically qualify for Extra Help because of any of these: • You have both Medicare and Medicaid • You're in a Medicare Savings Program • You get Supplemental Security Income (SSI) benefits	Purple	"Deemed Status Notice"
Automatically qualify for Extra Help because you qualify for Medicare and Medicaid **and** currently get benefits through Original Medicare	Yellow	"Auto-Enrollment Notice"
Continue to **automatically** qualify for Extra Help, but you'll have different copayment levels next year	Orange	"Change in Extra Help Copayment Notice"
Qualify for Extra Help because of one of these: • You belong to a Medicare Savings Program • You get Supplemental Security Income (SSI) • You applied and qualified for Extra Help	Green	"Facilitated Enrollment Notice"
Already get Extra Help, you joined a Medicare Prescription Drug Plan on your own, and your plan's premium is changing	Tan	"LIS Choosers Notice"
Already get Extra Help and Medicare reassigned you into a new Medicare Prescription Drug Plan for the coming year	Blue	"Reassign Formulary Notice"
No longer automatically qualify for Extra Help for the coming year	Grey	"Loss of Deemed Status Notice"

Visit Medicare.gov/forms-help-and-resources/mail-about-medicare/mail-about-medicare.html for more information about each type of letter.

How to Get Extra Help

Words in red are defined on pages 83–86.

If you automatically qualify for Extra Help, you don't need to apply.

Medicare mails **purple** "Deemed Status Notices" to people who automatically qualify for Extra Help. If you get one, keep it as proof that you qualify. You don't need to apply for Extra Help if you get this purple notice.

You automatically qualify for Extra Help if you get any of these:

- Full coverage from a state Medicaid program
- Help from your state Medicaid program paying your Medicare Part B premiums through a Medicare Savings Program
- Supplemental Security Income (SSI) benefits

If you aren't already in a Medicare drug plan, you must join one to get this Extra Help. If you don't join a Medicare drug plan on your own, Medicare will enroll you in a plan, unless you have certain retiree drug coverage from a former employer or union. If Medicare enrolls you in a plan, then Medicare will send you a **yellow** "Auto-Enrollment Notice" (if you get full Medicaid coverage) or a **green** "Facilitated Enrollment Notice" (if you belong to a Medicare Savings Program or get SSI) letting you know when your coverage begins. Check to see if the plan covers the drugs you use and if you can go to the pharmacies you want.

If Medicare enrolls you in a plan that doesn't meet your needs, you can switch plans at any time, and your new plan will begin the first day of the next month. If you don't want Medicare to enroll you in a Medicare drug plan, call the plan listed in the notice. Tell them you don't want to be in a Medicare drug plan and want to "opt out" of (decline) enrollment. Or, call 1-800-MEDICARE (1-800-633-4227). TTY users should call 1-877-486-2048.

How to Get Extra Help

Medicare drug plan costs if you **automatically qualify** for Extra Help in 2016

If you have Medicare and...	Your monthly premium*	Your yearly deductible	Your cost per drug at the pharmacy (until $4,850**)	Your cost per drug at the pharmacy (after $4,850**)
Full Medicaid coverage for each full month you live in an institution, like a nursing home	$0	$0	$0	$0
Full Medicaid coverage, and you get home- and community-based services	$0	$0	$0	$0
Full Medicaid coverage and have a yearly income at or below $11,880 (single) or $16,020 (married)	$0	$0	**Generic and certain preferred drugs:** No more than $1.20 **Brand-name drugs:** No more than $3.60	$0
Full Medicaid coverage and have a yearly income above $11,880 (single) or $16,020 (married)	$0	$0	**Generic and certain preferred drugs:** No more than $2.95 **Brand-name drugs:** No more than $7.40	$0
Help from Medicaid paying your Medicare Part B premiums	$0	$0	**Generic and certain preferred drugs:** No more than $2.95 **Brand-name drugs:** No more than $7.40	$0
Supplemental Security Income (SSI)	$0	$0	**Generic and certain preferred drugs:** No more than $2.95 **Brand-name drugs:** No more than $7.40	$0

Notes: *There are plans you can join and pay no premium. There are other plans where you'll have to pay part of the premium even when you automatically qualify for Extra Help. Tell your plan you qualify for Extra Help and ask how much you'll pay for your monthly premium.

** Your cost per drug generally decreases once the amount you pay and Medicare pays in Extra Help reaches $4,850 per year.

The cost sharing, income levels, and resources listed are for 2016 and can increase each year.
Income levels are higher if you live in Alaska or Hawaii, or you or your spouse pays at least half of the living expenses of dependent family members who live with you, or you work.

3

How to Get Extra Help

If you apply and qualify for Extra Help

If you think you qualify for Extra Help, you can do one of these:

- Visit socialsecurity.gov/i1020 to apply online, or call Social Security at 1-800-772-1213. TTY users should call 1-800-325-0778.

- Apply at your State Medical Assistance (Medicaid) office.

- Visit Medicare.gov/contacts, or call 1-800-MEDICARE (1-800-633-4227), and say "Medicaid" to get the phone number. TTY users should call 1-877-486-2048.

Words in red are defined on pages 83–86.

There's no risk or cost to apply. Remember, even if you qualify, you still need to join a Medicare drug plan to get the Extra Help. For more information on what income and resources count when you apply, see pages 39–40.

If you apply and qualify for Extra Help, in most cases Medicare will enroll you in a Medicare drug plan if you don't join one on your own. This makes sure you get help paying for your drug costs. Medicare will mail you a **green** letter letting you know when your coverage begins. Check to see if the plan covers the drugs you use and if you can go to the pharmacies you want. If not, you can change plans. If Medicare enrolls you in a plan that doesn't meet your needs, you can switch plans at any time, and your new plan will begin the first day of the next month.

If you don't want Medicare to enroll you in a Medicare drug plan (for example, because you want to keep your employer or union coverage), call the plan listed in the green letter. Tell them you don't want to be in a Medicare drug plan and want to "opt out" of (decline) enrollment. Or, call 1-800-MEDICARE.

3 How to Get Extra Help

Medicare drug plan costs if you **apply and qualify** for Extra Help in 2016

If you have Medicare and...	Your monthly premium*	Your yearly deductible	Your cost per drug at the pharmacy (until $4,850**)	Your cost per drug at the pharmacy (after $4,850**)
A yearly income below $16,038 (single) or $21,627 (married) with resources of no more than $8,780 (single) or $13,930 (married)	$0	$0	**Generic and certain preferred drugs:** No more than $2.95 **Brand-name drugs:** No more than $7.40	$0
A yearly income below $16,038 (single) or $21,627 (married) with resources between $8,780 – $13,640 (single) or $13,930 – $27,250 (married)	$0	$74	Up to 15% of the cost of each drug	**Generic and certain preferred drugs:** No more than $2.95 **Brand-name drugs:** No more than $7.40
A yearly income between $16,038 – $16,632 (single) or $21,627 – $22,428 (married) with resources up to $13,640 (single) or $27,250 (married)	25%	$74	Up to 15% of the cost of each drug	**Generic and certain preferred drugs:** No more than $2.95 **Brand-name drugs:** No more than $7.40
A yearly income between $16,632 – $17,226 (single) or $22,428 – $23,229 (married) with resources up to $13,640 (single) or $27,250 (married)	50%	$74	Up to 15% of the cost of each drug	**Generic and certain preferred drugs:** No more than $2.95 **Brand-name drugs:** No more than $7.40
A yearly income between $17,226 – $17,820 (single) or $23,229 – $24,030 (married) with resources up to $13,640 (single) or $27,250 (married)	75%	$74	Up to 15% of the cost of each drug	**Generic and certain preferred drugs:** No more than $2.95 **Brand-name drugs:** No more than $7.40

See the notes below the table on page 36 for more information.

How to Get Extra Help

How do I apply for Extra Help?

Whose income and resources count?

- **Your** own income and resources count.
- If you're married and live with your spouse, **both** of your incomes and resources count, even if only one of you applies for Extra Help.
- If you're married and don't live with your spouse when you apply, only **your** income and resources count.

Words in red are defined on pages 83–86.

Note: Married couples living together who both apply for Extra Help through Social Security can use the same application (SSA-1020), available at socialsecurity.gov/i1020.

What income counts?

"Income" means any cash, goods, or services you can use to meet your needs for food or shelter. Examples include (but aren't limited to):

Income counted	Income not counted
- Wages	- Supplemental Nutrition Assistance Program (SNAP)
- Earnings from self-employment	- Housing assistance
- Social Security benefits	- Home energy assistance
- Railroad Retirement benefits	- Medical treatment and drugs
- Veterans' benefits	- Disaster assistance
- Pensions	- Earned income tax credit payments
- Annuities	- Assistance from others to pay for household expenses
- Alimony	- Victim's compensation payments
- Rental income	- Scholarships and education grants
- Worker's compensation	

3

How to Get Extra Help

What resources count?

Social Security or your state must count your resources to decide if you qualify for Extra Help. Resources include the value of the things you own. Your resources include cash and other things you normally can convert to cash within 20 workdays. Examples include (but aren't limited to):

Resources counted

- Cash at home or anywhere else
- Bank accounts (checking, savings, and certificates of deposit)
- Stocks, bonds, savings bonds, mutual funds, Individual Retirement Accounts (IRA), or other similar investments
- Value of real estate **other** than your primary residence (the home you live in)

Resources not counted

- Your primary residence (the home you live in) and the land it's on
- Your personal possessions
- Your car(s) or vehicle(s)
- Things you couldn't easily convert to cash, like jewelry or furniture
- Burial expenses, burial plots, and interest earned on money you plan to use for burial expenses
- Life insurance policies
- Property needed for self-support, like rental property or land used to grow produce for home consumption
- Certain other money you're holding isn't counted for 9 months, like housing assistance

You should contact Social Security at 1-800-772-1213 to find out which other types of income and resources count and which are excluded. TTY users should call 1-800-325-0778.

How to Get Extra Help

How long will I get Extra Help if I qualify?

If you automatically qualify for Extra Help

To automatically qualify for Extra Help for the coming year, you must continue to qualify for Medicaid, get help from your state Medicaid program to pay Medicare Part B premiums (in a Medicare Savings Program), or get Supplemental Security Income (SSI).

If you won't automatically qualify the next year, you'll get a notice (on **grey** paper) in the mail by early fall. If the amount of Extra Help you get is changing, so that your copayment amounts change for next year, you'll get a notice (on **orange** paper) in the mail with the new copayment amounts. If you don't get a notice, you'll get the same level of Extra Help next year that you have this year.

Even if you get the notice on grey paper because you don't automatically qualify, you may still be able to save on your Medicare drug coverage costs. **You need to apply for Extra Help to find out.**

Words in red are defined on pages 83–86.

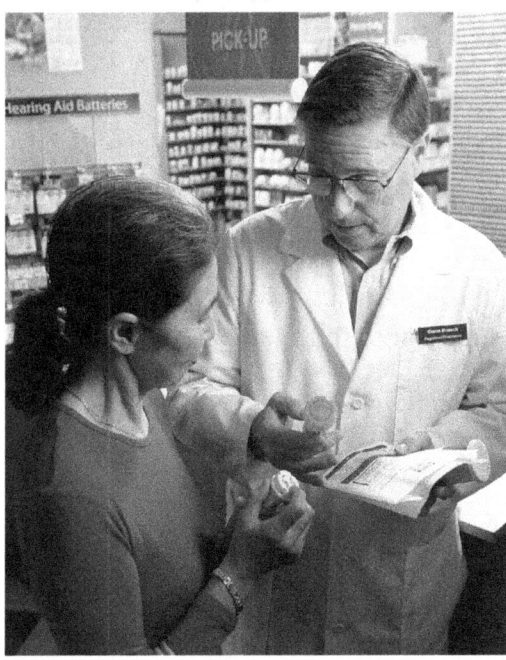

How to Get Extra Help

Words in red are defined on pages 83–86.

If you apply and qualify for Extra Help

If you qualify for Extra Help, you'll get the Extra Help for the calendar year as long as you're enrolled in a Medicare drug plan **and** there aren't changes to your income, resources, or family size.

You'll also get the Extra Help for the calendar year as long as you don't have a change in your marital status, like:

- Marriage
- Divorce
- Annulment
- Separation (not temporary)
- Spouses resume living together after separating
- Death of spouse (in this situation, the change in your Extra Help may be delayed for one year)

If you applied to Social Security for Extra Help and you qualified, notify them if your marital status changes, because it could raise, lower, or stop the amount of Extra Help you get. The change in Extra Help you get starts the month after you report the change in your marital status.

You can report changes in your income, resources, or family size to Social Security to review at any time. Any changes affecting your Extra Help start January 1 of the following year.

If you applied and qualified for Extra Help through your state, your state's rules may require you to tell them about changes in your circumstances.

3

How to Get Extra Help

If I qualify for Extra Help, what can I do to make sure I pay the right amount?

If you automatically qualify, you should get a **purple, yellow, orange,** or **green** notice from Medicare that you can show to your plan as proof you qualify for Extra Help (see chart on page 34). If you applied for Extra Help, you can show your plan your "Notice of Award" letter from Social Security as proof you qualify. If you have Supplemental Security Income (SSI), you can use your award letter from Social Security as proof you have SSI.

You can also give your plan any of the documents below as proof. Each item must show you were eligible for Medicaid during a month after June 2015.

Proof you have Medicaid and live in an institution or get home- and community-based services	Other proof you have Medicaid
▪ A bill from an institution (like a nursing home) or a copy of a state document showing Medicaid paid for your stay for at least a month ▪ A print out from your state's Medicaid system showing you lived in the institution for at least a month ▪ A document from your state that shows you have Medicaid and are getting home- and community-based services	▪ A copy of your Medicaid card (if you have one) ▪ A copy of a state document that shows you have Medicaid ▪ A print-out from a state electronic enrollment file, or screen print from your state's Medicaid systems that shows you have Medicaid ▪ Any other document from your state that shows you have Medicaid

Your plan must accept any of these documents as proof you qualify for Extra Help. As soon as you have given them any one of these documents, your plan must make sure you pay no more than the right amount to fill your prescriptions.

How to Get Extra Help

If you qualify for Extra Help because you have Medicaid, but you don't have or can't find any of these documents, ask your plan for help. Your plan must also contact Medicare so Medicare can get proof that you qualify, if it's available. You should expect your request to take anywhere from several days to up to 2 weeks, depending on the circumstances. Be sure to tell your plan how many days of medication you have left. Your plan and Medicare will work to process your request before you run out of medication, if possible.

If you paid for prescription drugs since you qualified for Extra Help, you may be able to get back part of what you paid. Keep your receipts, and call Medicare's Limited Income Newly Eligible Transition (NET) Program at 1-800-783-1307 for more information. TTY users should call 711.

If your plan doesn't correct a problem to help you pay the right amount for your drugs, doesn't respond to your request for help, or takes longer than expected to get back to you, call 1-800-MEDICARE (1-800-633-4227) to file a complaint. TTY users should call 1-877-486-2048.

What if my application for Extra Help is denied?

You have the right to appeal the decision. If you applied for Extra Help through Social Security, they'll give you a hearing by phone unless you choose a case review. Either way, Social Security will review those parts of the decision which you believe are wrong and will look at any new information you provide. Social Security may also review those parts which you believe are correct. Someone who wasn't involved in the first decision will decide your case.

How to Get Extra Help

To request an appeal, call Social Security at 1-800-772-1213. TTY users should call 1-800-325-0778. You can also get a copy of form SSA-1021 ("Appeal of Determination for Help with Medicare Prescription Drug Costs") and instructions on filling it out by visiting socialsecurity.gov/online.

If you want to file an appeal, keep in mind:

- You have 60 days to ask for an appeal.

- The 60 days start the day after you get a letter from Social Security denying your application. Social Security will assume you got the letter 5 days after the date on it, unless you show them you didn't get it within the 5-day period.

- You can have a lawyer, friend, or someone else help you. Call Social Security at 1-800-772-1213 for a list of groups that can help you with your appeal. To find your local Social Security office, visit socialsecurity.gov/locator.

If you apply for Extra Help **with your state, your decision letter should include appeal rights and procedures. Call your** State Medical Assistance (Medicaid) office **for information on your state's appeals process.** You can get the phone number for your state Medicaid office by visiting Medicare.gov/contacts, or by calling 1-800-MEDICARE (1-800-633-4227). TTY users should call 1-877-486-2048.

What if I don't qualify for Extra Help?

You can still choose and join a Medicare drug plan that meets your needs. You'll have to pay the monthly premium, yearly deductible (some plans don't have a deductible), and a share of the cost of your drugs.

Even if you don't qualify for Extra Help now, you can apply or reapply later if your income and resources change.

Your state may have programs to help you pay your prescription drug costs. Contact your state Medicaid office or State Health Insurance Assistance Program (SHIP) for more information. Visit shiptacenter.org or call 1-800-MEDICARE (1-800-633-4227) for the phone number of your SHIP. TTY users should call 1-877-486-2048.

Other ways to save if you don't get Extra Help

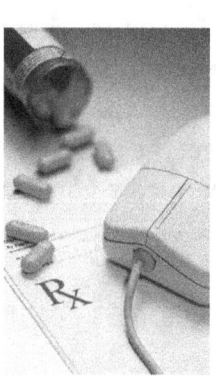

There are other ways you may also be able to save. Consider switching to drugs that cost less. Ask your doctor if there are generic, over-the-counter, or less-expensive brand-name drugs that could work just as well as the ones you're taking now. Switching to lower-cost drugs can save you hundreds or possibly thousands of dollars a year. Visit the Medicare Plan Finder at Medicare.gov/find-a-plan to get information on ways to save money in your Medicare drug plan.

How to Get Extra Help

You can also help lower your Medicare prescription drug costs by:

1. **Exploring National- and Community-Based Programs** that may have programs that can help you with your drug costs, like the National Patient Advocate Foundation or the National Organization for Rare Disorders. Get information on federal, state, and private assistance programs in your area by visiting benefitscheckup.org, the Benefits Check Up website. The help you get from some of these programs may count toward your true out-of-pocket (TrOOP) costs. TrOOP costs are the expenses that count toward your Medicare drug plan out-of-pocket expenses — up to $4,850 in 2016. These costs determine when your catastrophic coverage will begin.

2. **Looking at State Pharmaceutical Assistance Programs (SPAPs)** to see if you qualify. SPAPs in 21 states and 1 territory offer some type of coverage to help people with Medicare with paying drug plan premiums and/or cost sharing. Find out if your state has an SPAP at Medicare.gov/pharmaceutical-assistance-program/state-programs.aspx. See page 64 to find more information about SPAPs. SPAP contributions may count toward your TrOOP costs.

3. **Looking into Manufacturer's Pharmaceutical Assistance Programs (sometimes called Patient Assistance Programs (PAPs))** offered by the manufacturers of the drugs you take. Many of the major drug manufacturers offer assistance programs for people enrolled in a Medicare drug plan. Find out whether the manufacturers of the drugs you take offer a Pharmaceutical Assistance Program by visiting Medicare.gov/pharmaceutical-assistance-program. Assistance from PAPs isn't part of Medicare Part D, so any help you get from this type of program won't count toward your TrOOP costs.

3

How to Get Extra Help

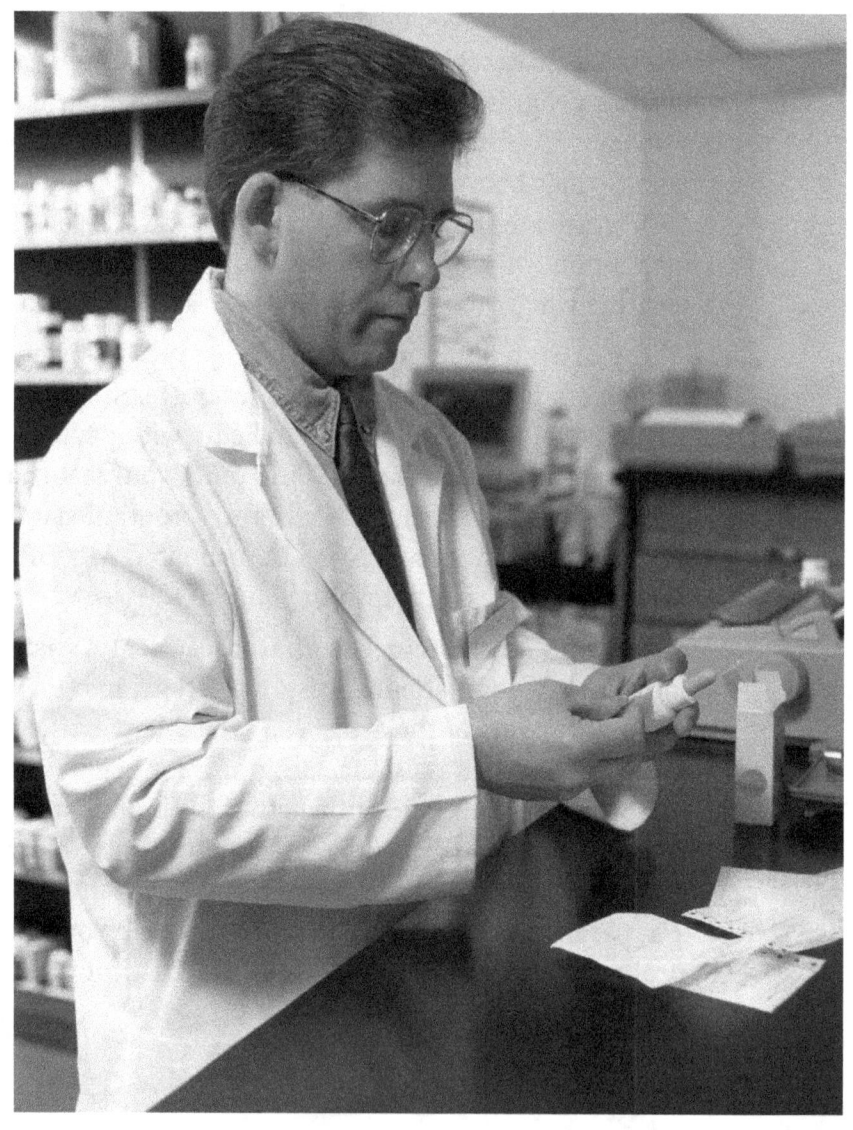

Your Coverage Choices

Read about the choices you have with Medicare drug coverage. **More than one situation may apply to you.**

Get help with drug coverage decisions

If you need help with your Medicare drug coverage decisions, call your State Health Insurance Assistance Program (SHIP). Visit shiptacenter.org, or call 1-800-MEDICARE (1-800-633-4227) to get the phone number of your SHIP. TTY users should call 1-877-486-2048.

Medicare works with other government representatives, community- and faith-based groups, employers and unions, doctors, pharmacies, and other people and organizations to educate people on drug coverage choices. Look for information in your local newspaper, or listen for information on the radio, about events in your community.

If you have limited income and resources, you may qualify for Extra Help paying the costs of Medicare drug coverage. See Section 3.

Words in red are defined on pages 83–86.

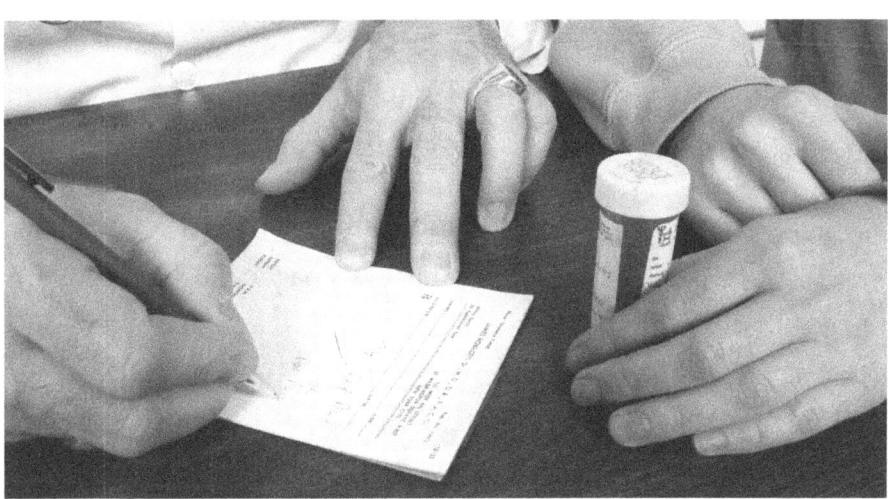

What else do I need to think about before I decide to get Medicare drug coverage?

Before you make a decision, get answers to these questions:

- Do I have creditable prescription drug coverage now?—In other words, if I have drug coverage, is it expected to pay, on average, at least as much as standard Medicare drug coverage? (Your current plan can tell you.)

- Should I keep my drug coverage, if I have coverage now?

- How will joining a Medicare drug plan and keeping my current drug coverage affect my current coverage? (Your current plan can tell you.)

- How would joining a particular Medicare drug plan affect my out-of-pocket costs?

- Would my premium be higher later if I wait to join a Medicare drug plan because I have to pay a late enrollment penalty? Would my coverage start when I want it to?

- Does a Medicare drug plan in my area cover the drugs I take? (Find out by visiting Medicare.gov/find-a-plan.)

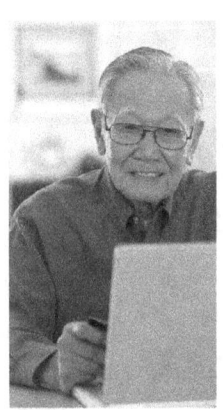

- Can I get Extra Help paying for my drug costs if I join a Medicare drug plan?

- Is there a particular pharmacy I want to use? Does it belong to a network of a Medicare drug plan in my area?

- Do I spend part of each year in another state? (This may be important if a plan you want to join requires you to use certain pharmacies.)

- What are a particular Medicare drug plan's quality ratings? (Compare Medicare Prescription Drug Plans at Medicare.gov/find-a plan.)

Words in red are defined on pages 83–86.

I have only Part A and/or Part B and no drug coverage

If you have Medicare Part A (Hospital Insurance) and/or Medicare Part B (Hospital Insurance) and live in a Medicare Prescription Drug Plan's service area, you can join that plan. Use the Medicare Plan Finder at Medicare.gov/find-a-plan or call 1-800-MEDICARE (1-800-633-4227) for a list of plans in your area. TTY users should call 1-877-486-2048. You can also look in your "Medicare & You" handbook. Not sure if you have Part A and/or Part B? Check your red, white, and blue Medicare card.

I have Medicare and a Medicare Supplement Insurance (Medigap) policy without drug coverage

You can join a Medicare drug plan by:

1. Keeping your current Medigap policy and enrolling in a Medicare Prescription Drug Plan.

2. Joining a Medicare Advantage Plan (like an HMO or PPO) in your area that includes drug coverage. You would get all your health care benefits and drug coverage from the plan.

> **If you join a Medicare Advantage Plan, you don't need a Medigap policy. If you already have a Medigap policy, you can't use it to pay for out-of-pocket costs under your Medicare Advantage Plan.** You may want to drop your Medigap policy if you join a Medicare Advantage Plan. However, you might not be able to get the same Medigap policy back if you leave the Medicare Advantage Plan and then go back to Original Medicare, or you may end up paying higher premiums for the Medigap policy.

You have a legal right to keep your Medigap policy, but rights to buy a Medigap policy may vary by state. For more information about your Medigap policy, contact your Medigap insurer or visit Medicare.gov.

If you're joining a Medicare Advantage Plan for the first time, you may get a 12-month trial period during which you can disenroll from the Medicare Advantage Plan and get back your Medigap policy, or if it isn't available, buy another Medigap policy.

4 Your Coverage Choices

Words in red are defined on pages 83–86.

I have Medicare and a Medicare Supplement Insurance (Medigap) policy with drug coverage

Before 2006, some Medigap policies included prescription drug coverage. If you still have a Medigap policy with drug coverage, your Medigap insurer must send you a detailed notice each year describing your choices for drug coverage and stating whether its drug coverage is creditable prescription drug coverage. Some of your choices for drug coverage include:

- Joining a Medicare Prescription Drug Plan and keeping your current Medigap policy without the drug coverage.

- Joining a Medicare Advantage Plan (like an HMO or PPO) that includes drug coverage. You would get all your health care coverage including drug coverage from this plan, and you wouldn't need a Medigap policy. If you join a Medicare Medical Savings Account (MSA) Plan (a type of Medicare Advantage Plan), you can continue to use your Medigap drug coverage, since MSAs can't offer Medicare drug coverage.

- Keeping your current Medigap policy with the drug coverage included.

Information you get from your Medigap insurer describes these choices in detail. You can also check with your State Insurance Department to find out what other options you may have for drug coverage. Visit Medicare.gov/contacts or call 1-800-MEDICARE (1-800-633-4227) to get the number of your State Insurance Department. TTY users should call 1-877-486-2048.

Tip: Contact your Medigap insurer before you make any changes to your drug coverage.

Your Coverage Choices

If you decide to join a Medicare Prescription Drug Plan, you can keep your current Medicare Supplemental Insurance (Medigap) policy without the drug coverage. You'll need to tell your Medigap insurer when your Medicare drug coverage starts. They must remove the drug coverage from your Medigap policy and adjust your premium based on this change. **Also, you may have to pay a late enrollment penalty to join a Medicare Prescription Drug Plan if the drug coverage you've had under your Medigap policy isn't creditable prescription drug coverage.** You may have to pay this higher premium for as long as you're in a Medicare Prescription Drug Plan.

For more information about Medigap policies, visit Medicare.gov or call 1-800-MEDICARE (1-800-633-4227). TTY users should call 1-877-486-2048. You can also call your State Health Insurance Assistance Program (SHIP) for more information about Medigap. Visit shiptacenter.org or call 1-800-MEDICARE to get the phone number of your SHIP.

I have Medicare and get drug coverage from a current or former employer or union

Before making a decision about whether to join a Medicare drug plan, find out how your employer or union drug coverage works with Medicare, because your coverage may change if you join a Medicare drug plan. Your employer or union (or the plan that administers your drug coverage) will send you a "Creditable Coverage" disclosure each year, letting you know if it's creditable prescription drug coverage and how it compares to Medicare drug coverage. Read carefully, and save all materials from your employer or union to know your options. If you don't get this information, ask your employer or union for it.

There are 3 times when you may have to make choices about your employer/union drug coverage and Medicare drug coverage:

3. During your 7-month Initial Enrollment Period, when you first become eligible for Medicare (see page 18 for details)

4. During Open Enrollment, between October 15–December 7 each year

5. When your employer/union coverage changes or ends

I have Medicare and get drug coverage from a current or former employer or union (continued)

Some important questions to answer before making a decision:

- Is your employer or union drug coverage creditable (on average, does it expect to pay at least as much as standard Medicare drug coverage)? If not, in most cases, you'll have to pay a late enrollment penalty if you don't join a Medicare drug plan when you're first eligible.

- Will you or your spouse or dependents lose all of your employer or union health coverage if you join a Medicare drug plan?

- How do out-of-pocket drug costs with your employer or union drug coverage compare to out-of-pocket drug costs with a Medicare drug plan?

- How will your costs change if you get Extra Help with your Medicare drug plan costs?

If your (or your spouse's) employer or union tells you your current coverage IS creditable prescription drug coverage:

- You can keep this coverage as long as your employer or union still offers it.

- You won't have to pay a late enrollment penalty if your employer or union stops offering drug coverage, or stops offering creditable prescription drug coverage, as long as you join a Medicare drug plan within 63 days after the coverage ends.

Note: Keep materials your employer or union sends you that tell you your drug coverage is creditable. You may need to show it to your Medicare drug plan as proof of creditable prescription drug coverage if you decide to join a Medicare drug plan later.

4 Your Coverage Choices

If your (or your spouse's) employer or union tells you your current coverage ISN'T creditable prescription drug coverage:

If you want to join a Medicare drug plan, in most cases you must join when you're first eligible to avoid a late enrollment penalty. If you don't enroll when you're first eligible, you may have to wait to join a Medicare drug plan until Open Enrollment, which is October 15–December 7.

Find out about your options from your benefits administrator. You may be able to do one of these:

- Keep your current employer or union drug coverage, and join a Medicare drug plan to get more complete drug coverage.

- Keep only your current employer or union drug coverage. If you join a Medicare drug plan later, you may have to pay a late enrollment penalty if your current drug coverage isn't creditable.

- Drop your current coverage and join a Medicare drug plan, or join a Medicare health plan that covers prescription drugs.

Words in red are defined on pages 83–86.

Caution: If you drop your employer or union coverage, you may not be able to get it back. You also may not be able to drop your employer or union **drug** coverage without also dropping your employer or union **health** coverage. If you drop coverage for yourself, you may also have to drop coverage for your spouse and dependents. Medicare doesn't have information about how your current employer or union drug coverage will be affected by your enrollment in a Medicare drug plan, so talk to your employer or union's benefits administrator before you make any decisions about your drug coverage.

Your Coverage Choices

I have Medicare and a Federal Employee Health Benefits (FEHB) plan

- During Open Enrollment, you'll get information about your drug coverage and whether it's creditable prescription drug coverage. Read this information carefully.

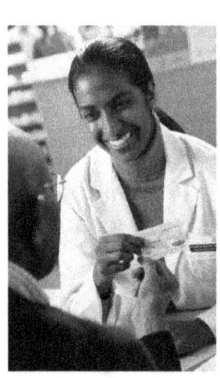

- Contact your FEHB insurer before making any changes. It'll almost always be to your advantage to keep your current coverage without any changes. It isn't cost effective for most people covered under a FEHB plan to join a Medicare drug plan unless they qualify for Extra Help. **Caution:** You can't drop FEHB drug coverage without also dropping FEHB plan coverage for hospital and medical services, which may mean higher costs for these services.

- If you qualify for Extra Help paying Medicare drug costs, see how your costs with a Medicare drug plan and any Extra Help would compare to your FEHB plan drug coverage.

- If you ever lose your FEHB coverage and need to join a Medicare drug plan, in most cases you won't have to pay a late enrollment penalty, if you join within 63 days of losing FEHB coverage.

- If you join a Medicare drug plan, you can keep your FEHB plan. In most cases, your Medicare drug plan pays first.

For more information, visit opm.gov/healthcare-insurance/healthcare or call the Office of Personnel Management at 1-888-767-6738. TTY users should call 1-800-878-5707. You can also call your plan.

Your Coverage Choices

I have Medicare and TRICARE or benefits from the Department of Veterans Affairs (VA) that include drug coverage

Words in red are defined on pages 83–86.

- As long as you still qualify, you can keep your TRICARE or VA drug coverage. TRICARE or your VA provider should send you information each year about your coverage and whether it's creditable prescription drug coverage. Read this information carefully, and save these materials.

- Before making any changes, contact your benefits administrator for information about your TRICARE or VA coverage. It's almost always to your advantage to keep your current coverage without any changes. For most people with TRICARE or VA coverage, unless you qualify for Extra Help, it isn't cost effective to join a Medicare drug plan.

- If you qualify for Extra Help paying Medicare drug costs, compare costs with a Medicare drug plan and any Extra Help to costs with your TRICARE or VA drug coverage.

- If you ever lose your TRICARE or VA coverage and need to join a Medicare drug plan, in most cases, you won't have to pay a late enrollment penalty, if you join within 63 days of losing TRICARE or VA coverage.

- If you join a Medicare drug plan and have VA coverage, you can't use both types of coverage for the same prescription.

- If you have TRICARE and join a Medicare Prescription Drug Plan, your Medicare Prescription Drug Plan pays first, and TRICARE pays second.

- If you join a Medicare Advantage Plan (like an HMO or PPO) with drug coverage, you must get prescription drugs through the Medicare Advantage Plan. The Medicare Advantage Plan is the primary payer. TRICARE may cover some or all of the claim unpaid by the Medicare Advantage Plan if the plan's pharmacy is a TRICARE network pharmacy that participates in the online coordination of benefits.

For more information on VA benefits, visit va.gov/healthbenefits, call the VA Health Benefits Service Center at 1-877-222-VETS (1-877-222-8387), or visit your local VA medical facility.

Get answers on how TRICARE works with Medicare drug coverage by calling the TRICARE Pharmacy Program at 1-877-363-1303. TTY users should call 1-877-540-6261.

Your Coverage Choices

I have a Medicare health plan without drug coverage

If you have a Medicare Advantage Plan (like an HMO or PPO) or another Medicare health plan that doesn't include drug coverage, you may want to think about other ways to get Medicare drug coverage.

- See if your current Medicare Advantage Plan offers a Medicare prescription drug option. If so, you can switch to that option.

- If your current plan doesn't offer Medicare drug coverage, you can switch to another Medicare health plan in your area that offers it.

- If your current plan doesn't offer Medicare drug coverage, you can switch to Original Medicare and join a Medicare Prescription Drug Plan.

Words in red are defined on pages 83–86.

- Only some Medicare Private Fee-for-Service (PFFS) Plans offer Medicare drug coverage. If your Medicare PFFS Plan doesn't offer Medicare drug coverage, you can join a Medicare Prescription Drug Plan to get this coverage.

- Medicare Medical Savings Account (MSA) Plans **don't** offer Medicare drug coverage. If you have a Medicare MSA Plan, you can join a Medicare Prescription Drug Plan to get drug coverage.

  - If you have a Medicare MSA Plan and a Medicare Prescription Drug Plan, any money you use from your MSA Plan account on Medicare drug plan deductibles or cost sharing counts toward your drug plan out-of-pocket costs. See pages 13–16.

  - If you have a Medicare MSA Plan and **don't** have a Medicare Prescription Drug Plan, you can use money in your MSA account for prescription or non-prescription drugs. These expenses don't count towards the MSA Plan deductible.

- If your Medicare Cost Plan doesn't offer Medicare drug coverage, you can join a separate Medicare Prescription Drug Plan to add drug coverage.

Your Coverage Choices

If you stay in a plan that doesn't offer drug coverage and you don't join a Medicare Prescription Drug Plan or have other creditable prescription drug coverage, you may have to pay a late enrollment penalty if you want Medicare drug coverage later.

Contact your plan for more information about your choices.

I have a Medicare health plan with drug coverage

If you have drug coverage from a Medicare Advantage Plan (like an HMO or PPO) or other Medicare health plan, in most cases, you'll need to get your Medicare drug coverage from your plan.

- If you're in a Medicare Advantage Plan and you join a Medicare drug plan, in most cases, you'll be disenrolled from your Medicare Advantage Plan and returned to Original Medicare.

- If you're in a Medicare Private Fee-for-Service (PFFS) Plan that doesn't offer Medicare drug coverage, you can join a separate Medicare drug plan to add drug coverage.

- With a Medicare Cost Plan, you can either get your Medicare drug coverage from the plan (if offered), or you can join a separate Medicare drug plan to add drug coverage.

Contact your plan for more information about your choices.

Your Coverage Choices

I have Medicare and Medicaid

Words in red are defined on pages 83–86.

Medicare helps pay for your prescription drugs instead of Medicaid. Because you have Medicaid, Medicare automatically gives you Extra Help with your Medicare drug plan costs. See pages 33–34 for information about your costs. If you live in an institution (like a nursing home), in most cases, you pay nothing for your covered drugs.

If you haven't joined a Medicare drug plan, Medicare will enroll you in a drug plan to make sure you have drug coverage (unless you already have certain retiree drug coverage). Medicare sends you a **yellow** notice telling you what drug plan you're in and when your coverage starts. Check to see if the plan covers the drugs you take and includes the pharmacies you use. You can switch to a different Medicare drug plan at any time.

If you filled any covered prescriptions before your Medicare drug plan coverage started, you may be able to get back some of the money you spent. Call Medicare's Limited Income Newly Eligible Transition (NET) Program at 1-800-783-1307 for more information. TTY users should call 711.

If you don't want Medicare drug coverage and you don't want Medicare to enroll you in a Medicare drug plan (for example, because you have other creditable prescription drug coverage), call 1-800-MEDICARE (1-800-633-4227) and tell them you want to "opt out" of (decline) Medicare drug coverage. TTY users should call 1-877-486-2048.

Caution: If you call 1-800-MEDICARE and opt out of a Medicare drug plan, you could be left without any drug coverage. You can change your mind and join a Medicare drug plan at any time without paying a late enrollment penalty as long as you continue to qualify for Extra Help.

In limited cases, some state Medicaid programs may pay for drugs Medicare doesn't cover. If you continue to qualify for Medicaid, Medicaid will still cover the other health care costs that Medicare doesn't cover. If you aren't sure whether you still qualify for Medicaid, call your State Medical Assistance (Medicaid) office. To get the phone number, visit Medicare.gov/contacts, or call 1-800-MEDICARE.

I have Medicare and get Supplemental Security Income (SSI) benefits or belong to a Medicare Savings Program

If you have Medicare and get SSI or belong to a Medicare Savings Program, Medicare will send you a **purple** notice letting you know you automatically qualify for Extra Help paying your Medicare drug coverage costs. You get it automatically when you join a Medicare drug plan. See pages 33–34 for more information about your costs.

If you don't join a Medicare drug plan on your own, Medicare will enroll you in a Medicare Prescription Drug Plan, **to make sure you have coverage,** unless you already have certain retiree drug coverage. Medicare sends you a **yellow** or a **green** notice letting you know when your coverage begins. You can switch to a different Medicare drug plan at any time as long as you continue to qualify for Extra Help.

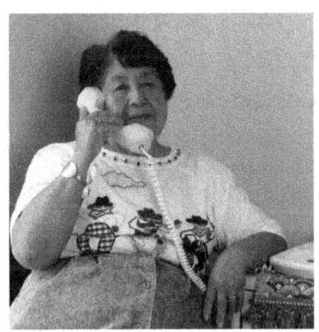
If you don't want Medicare drug coverage, and you don't want Medicare to enroll you in a Medicare drug plan (for example, because you have other creditable prescription drug coverage), call 1-800-MEDICARE (1-800-633-4227) and tell them you want to "opt out" of (decline) Medicare prescription drug coverage. TTY users should call 1-877-486-2048.

Caution: If you call 1-800-MEDICARE and tell them you don't want to join a Medicare drug plan, you could be left without drug coverage. You can change your mind and join a Medicare drug plan at any time without paying a late enrollment penalty as long as you continue to qualify for Extra Help.

I have Medicare and live in a nursing home or other institution

- **While you're living in an** institution, you can switch Medicare drug plans at any time.

- **If you move into or out of a nursing home or other institution,** you can switch Medicare drug plans at that time.

- **If you're in a skilled nursing facility getting Medicare-covered skilled nursing care,** Medicare Part A (Hospital Insurance) will generally cover your drugs.

- **If you live in a nursing home or other institution,** you'll get your covered drugs from a long-term care pharmacy that works with your Medicare drug plan. This long-term care pharmacy usually contracts with (or is owned and operated by) your institution.

Words in red are defined on pages 83–86.

Unless you choose a Medicare Advantage Plan (like an HMO or PPO) with drug coverage or a Medicare Prescription Drug Plan on your own, Medicare automatically enrolls people with both Medicare and full Medicaid coverage living in institutions into Medicare Prescription Drug Plans. If you live in a nursing home and have full Medicaid coverage, you pay nothing for your covered drugs after Medicaid has paid for your stay for at least one full calendar month.

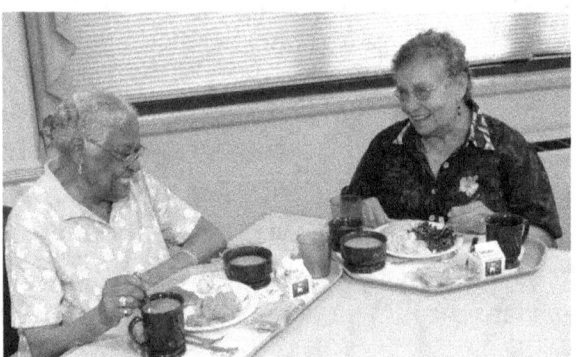

Note: Institutions don't include assisted living, adult living facilities, residential homes, or any kind of nursing home not certified by Medicare or Medicaid.

Your Coverage Choices

I have Medicare and benefits through Programs of All-inclusive Care for the Elderly (PACE)

Programs of All-inclusive Care for the Elderly (PACE) are a joint Medicare and Medicaid option in some states. PACE gives you your Medicare drug coverage, so you don't need to join a separate Medicare drug plan.

Caution: Joining a Medicare drug plan will disenroll you from your PACE plan. Your PACE plan gives you not only your drug coverage, but **all** of your health care services. If you join a Medicare drug plan, you'll become disenrolled from your PACE plan, and you'll no longer get other health care benefits through PACE. Contact your PACE plan for more information.

If you also have full Medicaid coverage, you get drugs at no cost to you through your PACE plan.

If you have Medicare only, you get all of your health care benefits, including drug coverage, through your PACE plan. You pay a reduced monthly PACE premium because it doesn't include prescription drugs. However, you'll also pay a separate Medicare prescription drug premium to your PACE organization or plan to cover the cost of your drugs.

If you don't have Medicaid coverage, you may still qualify for Extra Help paying for Medicare drug coverage. See Section 3 for more information about Extra Help.

I have Medicare and get help from my State Pharmacy Assistance Program (SPAP) paying drug costs

Words in red are defined on pages 83–86.

Several states have programs to help certain people pay for prescription drugs. Depending on your state, the State Pharmacy Assistance Program (SPAP) will have different ways to help you pay your drug costs. Some SPAPs may require you to join a Medicare drug plan, and then they'll cover the costs that Medicare doesn't cover. Find your SPAP's contact information by visiting Medicare.gov/pharmaceutical-assistance-program/state-programs.aspx. SPAP contributions count toward your true out-of-pocket (TrOOP) costs, the expenses that count toward your Medicare drug plan out-of-pocket threshold (or limit), which is $4,850 in 2016.

If you belong to an SPAP, you may have another opportunity each year to join a plan in addition to the October 15–December 7 Open Enrollment Period. You can switch one time in a calendar year to a different plan from the one your SPAP enrolled you in. If you lose your SPAP benefits, you're allowed to choose a different Medicare drug plan at any time during the month you lose your benefits and through the following 2 months.

Your SPAP will give you more information on how Medicare drug coverage affects the help you get now.

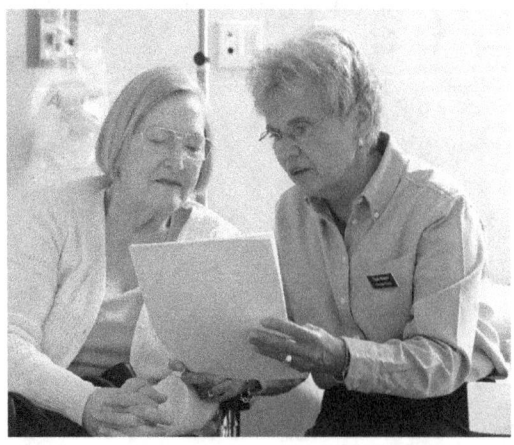

I get help from an AIDS Drug Assistance Program (ADAP)

Most AIDS Drug Assistance Programs (ADAPs) only cover HIV/AIDS-related medications. If they don't cover other drugs, they **aren't** creditable prescription drug coverage. If you don't have creditable prescription drug coverage and delay joining a Medicare drug plan, you may have to pay a late enrollment penalty to join later.

All Medicare drug plans cover all antiretroviral medications. Your ADAP may require you to join a Medicare drug plan to get ADAP benefits. An ADAP can cover Medicare drug plan premiums, deductibles, coinsurance, and/or copayments to help with your drug costs. Check with your ADAP to see if it requires you to join or if it'll help pay for these costs.

ADAPs vary by state so contact your ADAP to learn how it'll work with Medicare's drug coverage. ADAP contributions count toward your true out-of-pocket (TrOOP) costs, the expenses that count toward your Medicare drug plan out-of-pocket threshold (or limit), which is $4,850 in 2016.

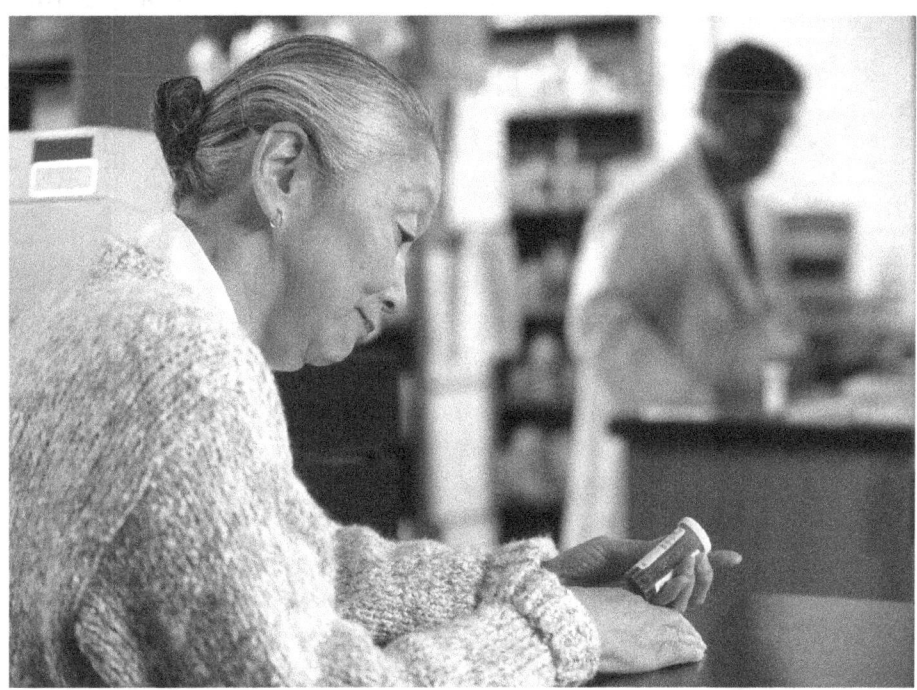

Your Coverage Choices

I have Medicare and get drug coverage from the Indian Health Service, Tribe or Tribal Health Organization, or Urban Indian Health Program

- You and your community may benefit if you join a Medicare drug plan. Ask your health provider or benefits coordinator if joining a plan is right for you. If you decide to join, they can help you find a plan.

- If you get prescription drugs through an Indian health pharmacy, you pay nothing.

- Joining a Medicare drug plan may be helpful to your Indian health provider because the drug plan pays part of the cost of your drugs. This helps the Indian health provider with the cost of services.

- If you have full coverage from Medicaid and live in a nursing home, you pay nothing for your Medicare drug coverage. See your Indian health provider or check with the benefits coordinator at your local Indian health pharmacy to get more information on how to join a plan.

Words in red are defined on pages 83–86.

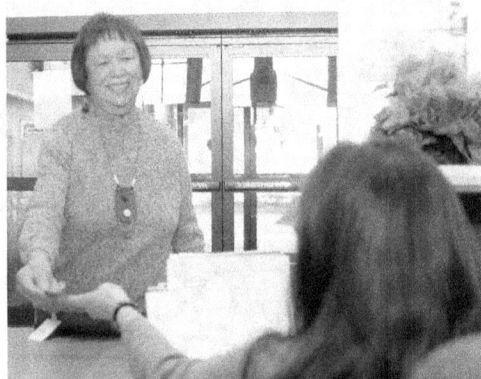

- If you get health care from the Indian Health Service, Tribal Health Program, or Urban Indian Health Program, you have creditable prescription drug coverage. You won't have to pay a penalty to join a Medicare drug plan later. Ask your Indian health care provider for a letter stating you have creditable prescription drug coverage.

3 Steps to Choosing a Medicare Drug Plan

Follow the steps below to choose and join a Medicare drug plan, whether you're joining for the first time or reviewing your plan options for coverage next year. Use the personal worksheets on pages 68–69 to help decide which plan meets your needs:

Step 1: Prepare—Gather information about your current drug coverage and needs.

Step 2: Compare—Compare Medicare drug plans based on cost, coverage, and customer service.

Step 3: Decide—Decide which plan is best for you, and join.

Tip: Before considering which Medicare drug plan to join, check out how any current health coverage you have could affect your drug coverage choices. See Section 4.

Step 1: Gather information about your current drug coverage and needs

Before choosing a Medicare drug plan, you may want to gather together some information about yourself. You need information about any drug coverage you may currently have, as well as a list of the drugs and doses you currently take. Also, gather any notices you get from Medicare, Social Security, or your current Medicare drug plan about changes to your plan.

If you have drug coverage, you need to find out whether it's creditable prescription drug coverage. Your current insurer or plan provider is required to notify you each year whether your coverage is creditable prescription drug coverage. If you haven't heard from your insurer or plan, call the insurer, your plan, or your benefits administrator to find out. Request a notice about whether your coverage is creditable prescription drug coverage if you didn't get one. Also, you may want to consider keeping your creditable prescription drug coverage rather than choosing a Medicare drug plan.

5

3 Steps to Choosing a Medicare Drug Plan

Drugs I take:

Drug name	Dosage (ml, mg)	Number of times a day I take my drug	Amount I pay each month

Today's date:_____

Step 2: Compare Medicare drug plans based on cost, coverage, and customer service

For lists of the specific drug plans available in your area, use the Medicare Plan Finder at Medicare.gov/find-a-plan, or call 1-800-MEDICARE (1-800-633-4227). TTY users should call 1-877-486-2048. You can also look in your "Medicare & You" handbook.

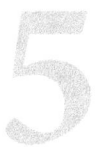

3 Steps to Choosing a Medicare Drug Plan

When you find some plans you're interested in, use Medicare.gov to get the information below, or call the companies that offer the plans directly.

Plan name:

Monthly premium $	Yearly deductible $	My drugs that are covered	My drugs that **aren't** covered	Amount I'd pay for each drug	Could I use my pharmacy?	Is mail order available?
		1.	1.			
		2.	2.			
		3.	3.			

Plan name:

Monthly premium $	Yearly deductible $	My drugs that are covered	My drugs that **aren't** covered	Amount I'd pay for each drug	Could I use my pharmacy?	Is mail order available?
		1.	1.			
		2.	2.			
		3.	3.			

Plan name:

Monthly premium $	Yearly deductible $	My drugs that are covered	My drugs that **aren't** covered	Amount I'd pay for each drug	Could I use my pharmacy?	Is mail order available?
		1.	1.			
		2.	2.			
		3.	3.			

3 Steps to Choosing a Medicare Drug Plan

Refer to the worksheets on pages 68–69. Compare the Medicare drug plans based on what's most important to your situation and your drug needs. You may want to ask yourself:

- Which plan(s) cover the drugs I take?
- Which plan gives me the best overall price on all of my drugs?
- What's the monthly premium, yearly deductible, and the coinsurance or copayment(s)?
- Which plan(s) allows me to use the pharmacy I want?
- Which plan(s) allows me to get drugs through the mail?
- Which plan(s) provides me with coverage in multiple states (if I need it)?
- What are the plans' quality ratings?
- Will I have to pay a penalty because I waited to join?
- Can my coverage start when I want it to?
- Is it likely that I'll need protection against unexpected drug costs in the future?
- If I already have a Medicare drug plan, am I satisfied with my plan's service?

If you need help with your Medicare drug coverage decisions, call your State Health Insurance Assistance Program (SHIP). Visit shiptacenter.org, or call 1-800-MEDICARE (1-800-633-4227) for the phone number of your SHIP. TTY users should call 1-877-486-2048.

Step 3: Decide which plan is best for you, and join

After you pick a plan that meets your needs, call the company offering it and ask how to join. You may be able to join by phone, by paper application, or online. You'll have to give the number on your Medicare card when you join.

Words in red are defined on pages 83–86.

Tips for Using Your New Medicare Drug Coverage

If you've just joined a Medicare Prescription Drug Plan (Part D) for the first time, or you switched to a new Medicare drug plan, there are some things you can do to make sure your first visit to the pharmacy goes smoothly.

The first time you use your new Medicare drug plan, you should come to the pharmacy with as much information as possible. Here's what you need to bring to the pharmacy:

- Your red, white, and blue Medicare card
- Photo ID (like a state driver's license or passport)
- Your plan membership card

If you don't have a plan membership card, you should also bring these to the pharmacy:

- An acknowledgement or confirmation letter from the plan, if you have one
- An enrollment confirmation number from the plan, if you have one (**Note:** Only confirmation numbers from the plan will work, not those from Medicare's Online Enrollment Center at Medicare.gov.)
- The name of the Medicare drug plan you joined (**Note:** If you haven't gotten a plan membership card or any plan enrollment materials, letting your pharmacist know the name of your plan can help them confirm your plan enrollment and get the information they need to bill your plan. The pharmacist may have to search for your plan information, and it may take extra time for them to fill your prescription.)

If you have both Medicare and Medicaid or qualify for Extra Help

If you have both Medicare and Medicaid or qualify for Extra Help with drug plan costs, you should also bring proof of your enrollment in Medicaid or proof that you qualify for Extra Help with you to the pharmacy. This is to help make sure you pay the right amount for your drugs. See the chart on page 34 for a list of some of the letters that prove you qualify for Extra Help.

Tips for Using Your New Medicare Drug Coverage

Proof of Medicaid **may include:**

- Your Medicaid card
- A copy of your current Medicaid award letter
- A copy of your yellow automatic enrollment letter from Medicare

Proof of Extra Help **may include:**

Words in red are defined on pages 83–86.

- A copy of your Medicaid card
- A copy of your **purple, yellow, orange, green, tan,** or **blue** Extra Help letter from Medicare (see chart on page 34)
- A copy of your Extra Help "Notice of Award" letter from Social Security
- A copy of your Supplemental Security Income (SSI) award letter
- Other proof that you qualify for Extra Help (like a "Notice of Award" letter from a state Medicaid program)

You don't need to have all of these items, but anything you can bring will help the pharmacist confirm your Medicare drug plan enrollment and/or that you qualify for Medicaid or Extra Help, to make sure you pay no more than the right amount to fill your prescriptions.

What if the pharmacist can't confirm my drug plan or Extra Help status?

In some rare cases, the pharmacist may not be able to confirm your plan enrollment or that you qualify for Medicaid or Extra Help. If this happens, your doctor may be able to give you a sample of your drug to help until your coverage is confirmed. You can also pay out-of-pocket for the drug. You should save the receipts and work with your new Medicare drug plan to get paid back for the drugs that would normally be covered under your plan.

If you paid for drugs out-of-pocket before you were enrolled in a Medicare drug plan but after you qualified for both Medicare and Medicaid or Supplemental Security Income (SSI), you may be able to get paid back for those costs. Call Medicare's Limited Income NET Program at 1-800-783-1307 to see if you qualify. TTY users should call 711.

Rights & Appeals

How do I protect myself from fraud and identity theft?

Help protect yourself by knowing whether Medicare Advantage Plans (like HMOs or PPOs) and Medicare Prescription Drug Plans are marketing to you properly. These plans and people who work with Medicare **aren't** allowed to:

- Charge you a fee to enroll in a plan.

- Send you unwanted emails.

- Come to your home uninvited to get you to join a Medicare plan.

- Call you, unless you're already a plan member. If you're a member, the agent who helped you join can call you.

- Offer you money to join their plan or give you free meals while trying to sell you a plan.

- Enroll you into a drug plan over the phone unless you call them and ask to enroll.

- Ask you for payment over the phone or online. The plan must send you a bill.

- Sell you a non-health related product, like an annuity or life insurance policy, while trying to sell you a Medicare health or drug plan.

- Make an appointment to tell you about their plan unless you agree (in writing or through a recorded phone discussion) to the products being discussed. During the appointment, they can only try to sell you the products you agreed to hear about.

- Talk to you about their plan in areas where you get health care, like an exam room, hospital patient room, or at a pharmacy counter.

- Try to sell you their plans or enroll you during an educational event, like a health fair or conference.

Independent agents and brokers working for plans must be licensed by the state. The plan must tell the state which agents are selling its plans.

Rights & Appeals

If you're in a Medicare drug plan and you think the plan may be breaking these rules, call the Medicare Drug Integrity Contractor (MEDIC) at 1-877-7SAFERX (1-877-772-3379).

Identity theft happens when someone uses your personal information without your permission to commit fraud or other crimes. Personal information includes things like your name, or your Social Security, Medicare, bank account, or credit card numbers.

Words in red are defined on pages 83–86.

If you think someone is misusing your personal information, call the Federal Trade Commission's ID Theft Hotline at 1-877-438-4338 to make a report. TTY users should call 1-866-653-4261. For more information about identity theft or to file a complaint online, visit consumer.gov/section/scams-and-identity-theft.

What if I need help applying for Extra Help, joining a Medicare drug plan, or requesting a coverage determination or appeal?

You may have a legal representative who, by state or federal law, has the legal right (like through a Power of Attorney or a court order) to act on your behalf. You can also appoint a family member, friend, advocate, attorney, doctor, or someone else to act as your representative.

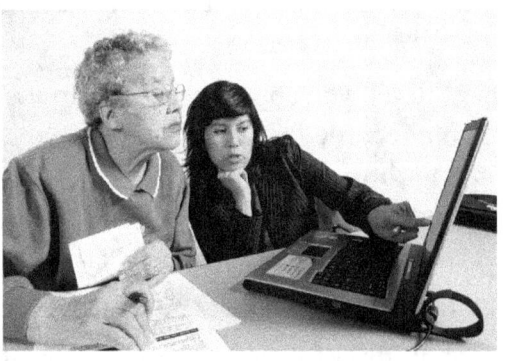

A representative can help you (or act on your behalf) apply to see if you qualify for Extra Help paying for Medicare drug coverage, or file a request for a coverage determination, complaint (also called a "grievance"), or appeal. Your doctor or other prescriber can request a coverage determination or first- or second-level appeal for you without being your appointed representative. **A representative can't enroll you in a Medicare drug plan unless they're also your legal representative according to the laws of your state.**

Rights & Appeals

A representative can be any of these:

- The person who acts on your behalf if you're incapacitated or can't make decisions for yourself.

- Anyone you choose to act as your representative (like your spouse, your child, or a caregiver).

- Your "representative payee" (sometimes called a "rep payee"). This is a person, agency, organization, or institution that Social Security selects to act on your behalf.

You can appoint your representative in one of these ways:

1. Fill out an "Appointment of Representative" form (CMS Form Number 1696) at Medicare.gov/MedicareOnlineForms, or call 1-800-MEDICARE (1-800-633-4227) and ask for a free copy. TTY users should call 1-877-486-2048.

2. Submit a letter that includes:

    —Your name, address, and phone number

    —Your Medicare number (found on your red, white, and blue Medicare card) or plan identification card

    —A statement appointing someone as your representative

    —The name, address, and phone number of your representative

    —The professional status of your representative or his or her relationship to you

    —A statement authorizing the release of your personal and identifiable health information to your representative

    —A statement explaining why you're being represented

    —Your signature and the date you signed the letter

    —Your representative's signature and the date he or she signed the letter

Rights & Appeals

Words in red are defined on pages 83–86.

Your representative must send the form or letter with your appeal request. See page 78 on how to request an appeal. The person helping you must send a copy of the form or letter each time you file a coverage determination or appeal, so keep a copy of everything you send to Medicare as part of your appeal. If you have questions about appointing a representative, call 1-800-MEDICARE (1-800-633-4227). TTY users should call 1-877-486-2048.

What if my enrollment in a Medicare drug plan is denied?

Medicare drug plans generally have to accept all eligible applicants who live in their service area, regardless of the applicant's age or health status. If your enrollment form is denied, the company will send you a letter explaining why. You may contact the plan for more information about your options.

What if my plan won't cover a drug I need?

If your Medicare drug plan won't cover a drug you think should be covered, or it will cover the drug at a higher cost than you think you should have to pay, you have these options:

1. Talk to your prescriber (the professional who wrote your prescription).

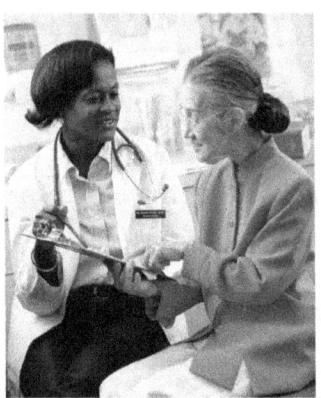

Ask your prescriber if you meet prior authorization or step therapy requirements. Contact your plan for more information on these requirements. You can also ask your prescriber if there are generic, over-the-counter, or less expensive brand-name drugs that could work just as well as the ones you're taking now.

2. Request a coverage determination (including an "exception").

You, your representative, your doctor, or other prescriber can request (orally or in writing) that your plan cover the drug you need. You can request a coverage determination if your pharmacist or plan tells you one of these:

- A drug you believe should be covered isn't covered.

- A drug is covered at a higher cost than you think you should have to pay.

- You have to meet a plan coverage rule (like prior authorization) before you can get the drug you requested.

- It won't cover a drug on the formulary because the plan believes you don't need the drug.

You, your representative, your doctor, or other prescriber can request a coverage determination called an "exception" if:

- You think your plan should cover a drug that's not on its formulary (drug list) because the other treatment options on your plan's formulary won't work for you.

- Your doctor or other prescriber believes you can't meet one of your plan's coverage rules, like prior authorization, step therapy, or quantity or dosage limits.

- You think your plan should charge a lower amount for a drug you're taking on the plan's non-preferred drug tier because the other treatment options in your plan's preferred drug tier won't work for you.

If you request an exception, your doctor or other prescriber will need to give a supporting statement to your plan explaining why you need the drug you're requesting. Check with your plan to find out if the supporting statement is required to be made in writing. The plan's decision-making time period begins once your plan gets the supporting statement.

You can either request a coverage determination before you pay for or get your drug, or you can decide to pay for the drug, save your receipt, and request that the plan pay you back by requesting a coverage determination.

Rights & Appeals

For details on filing a coverage determination, visit Medicare.gov/appeals.

If your plan denies your request, it will send you a letter explaining why the drug you requested isn't covered and instructions on how to file an appeal. If you disagree with the coverage determination decision, you have the right to appeal.

How do I appeal if I have Medicare drug coverage?

If you have Medicare drug coverage through a Medicare Prescription Drug Plan (PDP), a Medicare Advantage Plan with drug coverage (MA-PD), or other Medicare plan, your plan will send you information that explains your rights (called an "Evidence of Coverage" (EOC)). Call your plan if you have questions about your EOC.

Words in red are defined on pages 83–86.

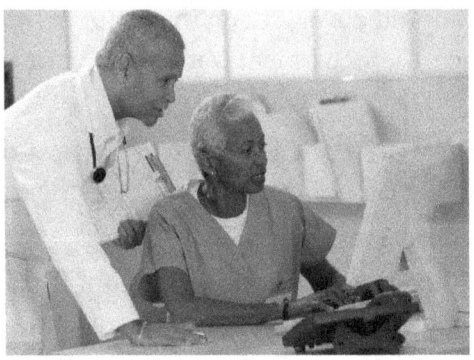

You have the right to ask your plan to provide or pay for a drug you think should be covered, provided, or continued. You have the right to request an appeal if you disagree with the plan's decision.

If you decide to appeal, ask your doctor or other prescriber for any information that may help your case. Keep a copy of everything you send to your plan as part of your appeal.

What's the appeals process for Medicare drug coverage?

The appeals process has 5 levels. If you disagree with the decision made at any level of the process, you can generally go to the next level. At each level, you'll be given instructions on how to move to the next level of appeal. For details on the appeals process, visit Medicare.gov/appeals.

How do I file a complaint (grievance)?

If you have a concern or a problem with your plan that isn't a request for coverage or reimbursement for a drug, you have the right to file a complaint (also called a "grievance").

Some examples of why you might file a complaint include:

- You believe your plan's customer service hours of operation should be different.
- You have to wait too long for your drug.
- The company offering your plan is sending you materials that you didn't ask to get and aren't related to the drug plan.
- The plan didn't make a timely decision about a coverage determination or didn't send your case to the Independent Review Entity (IRE) when it should have.
- You disagree with the plan's decision not to grant your request for an expedited (fast) coverage determination or first-level appeal (called a "redetermination").
- The plan didn't provide you with the required notices.
- The plan's notices don't follow Medicare rules.

If you want to file a complaint, you should know:

- You must file your complaint within 60 days from the date of the event that led to the complaint.
- You can file your complaint with the plan over the phone or in writing.
- You must be notified of the plan's decision generally no later than 30 days after the plan gets the complaint.
- If the complaint relates to a plan's refusal to make an expedited (fast) coverage determination or redetermination and you haven't yet purchased or received the drug, the plan must notify you of its decision within 24 hours after it gets the complaint.
- If you think you were charged too much for a drug, call the company offering your plan to get the most up-to-date price.

If the plan doesn't address your complaint, call 1-800-MEDICARE (1-800-633-4227). TTY users should call 1-877-486-2048.

More information on filing a complaint

- Visit Medicare.gov/appeals.

- Call your State Health Insurance Assistance Program (SHIP) for free, personalized counseling and help filing a complaint. To get the phone number of the SHIP in your state, visit shaptacenter.org or call 1-800-MEDICARE (1-800-633-4227). TTY users should call 1-877-486-2048.

What if I don't agree with Medicare's late enrollment penalty?

If you don't join a Medicare drug plan when you're first eligible, you may have to pay a late enrollment penalty unless you had other creditable prescription drug coverage. In some cases, you have the right to ask Medicare to review your late enrollment penalty. This is called a "reconsideration."

Some reasons why you may ask for a reconsideration include:

- You think Medicare didn't count all your previous creditable prescription drug coverage.

- You didn't get a notice that clearly explained whether your previous drug coverage was creditable.

Words in red are defined on pages 83–86.

Your Medicare drug plan will give you a reconsideration request form when it sends you the letter telling you that you have to pay a late enrollment penalty. Mail the completed form to the address, or fax it to the number listed on the form within 60 days from the date on the letter. You should also send any proof that supports your case, like information about previous creditable prescription drug coverage.

If you need more information about requesting a reconsideration of your late enrollment penalty, call your Medicare drug plan. You can also visit Medicare.gov, or call 1-800-MEDICARE (1-800-633-4227) for help. TTY users should call 1-877-486-2048.

For More Information

For more information about Medicare drug coverage, visit Medicare.gov/find-a-plan to get personalized information. Enter and save your current drug information to get more detailed cost information.

You also can call **1-800-MEDICARE** (1-800-633-4227) 24 hours a day, including weekends, to get information you need. TTY users should call 1-877-486-2048.

Note: If you want Medicare to give your personal health information to someone other than you, you need to let Medicare know in writing. You can fill out a "Medicare Authorization to Disclose Personal Health Information" form (CMS Form Number 10106) at Medicare.gov/MedicareOnlineForms, or call 1-800-MEDICARE (1-800-633-4227) to get a copy of the form. TTY users should call 1-877-486-2048.

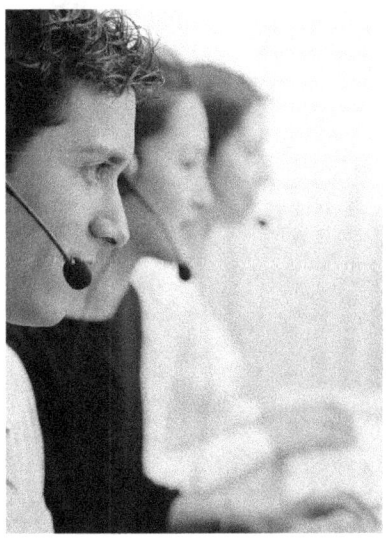

- **For more information about your current drug coverage,** contact your benefits administrator, insurer, or plan.

- **For more information about applying for** Extra Help **with your Medicare drug plan costs,** call Social Security at 1-800-772-1213, or visit socialsecurity.gov. TTY users should call 1-800-325-0778.

- **For free personalized counseling on your coverage choices,** contact your State Health Insurance Assistance Program (SHIP). Visit shiptacenter.org or call 1-800-MEDICARE (1-800-633-4227) for the phone number of your SHIP.

Definitions

Coinsurance—An amount you may be required to pay as your share of the cost for services after you pay any deductibles. Coinsurance is usually a percentage (for example, 20%).

Copayment—An amount you may be required to pay as your share of the cost for a medical service or supply, like a doctor's visit, hospital outpatient visit, or prescription drug. A copayment is usually a set amount, rather than a percentage. For example, you might pay $10 or $20 for a doctor's visit or prescription drug.

Coverage determination—The first decision made by your Medicare drug plan (not the pharmacy) about your drug benefits, including:

- Whether a particular drug is covered
- Whether you have met all the requirements for getting a requested drug
- How much you're required to pay for a drug
- Whether to make an exception to a plan rule when you request it

The drug plan must give you a prompt decision (72 hours for standard requests, 24 hours for expedited requests). If you disagree with the plan's coverage determination, the next step is an appeal.

Coverage gap (Medicare prescription drug coverage)—A period of time in which you pay higher cost sharing for prescription drugs until you spend enough to qualify for catastrophic coverage. The coverage gap (also called the "donut hole") starts when you and your plan have paid a set dollar amount for prescription drugs during that year.

Creditable prescription drug coverage—Prescription drug coverage (for example, from an employer or union) that's expected to pay, on average, at least as much as Medicare's standard prescription drug coverage. People who have this kind of coverage when they become eligible for Medicare can generally keep that coverage without paying a penalty, if they decide to enroll in Medicare prescription drug coverage later.

Deductible—The amount you must pay for health care or prescriptions before Original Medicare, your prescription drug plan, or your other insurance begins to pay.

Drug list—A list of prescription drugs covered by a prescription drug plan or another insurance plan offering prescription drug benefits. This list is also called a formulary.

Definitions

End-Stage Renal Disease (ESRD)—Permanent kidney failure that requires a regular course of dialysis or a kidney transplant.

Exception—A type of Medicare prescription drug coverage determination. A formulary exception is a drug plan's decision to cover a drug that's not on its drug list or to waive a coverage rule. A tiering exception is a drug plan's decision to charge a lower amount for a drug that is on its non-preferred drug tier. You or your prescriber can request an exception, and your doctor or other prescriber must provide a supporting statement explaining the medical reason for the exception.

Extra Help—A Medicare program to help people with limited income and resources pay Medicare prescription drug program costs, like premiums, deductibles, and coinsurance.

Institution—For the purposes of this publication, an institution is a facility that provides short-term or long-term care, such as a nursing home, skilled nursing facility (SNF), or rehabilitation hospital. Private residences, such as an assisted living facility or group home, aren't considered institutions for this purpose.

Medicaid—A joint federal and state program that helps with medical costs for some people with limited income and resources. Medicaid programs vary from state to state, but most health care costs are covered if you qualify for both Medicare and Medicaid.

Medically necessary—Health care services or supplies needed to diagnose or treat an illness, injury, condition, disease, or its symptoms and that meet accepted standards of medicine.

Medicare—Medicare is the federal health insurance program for people who are 65 or older, certain younger people with disabilities, and people with End-Stage Renal Disease (permanent kidney failure requiring dialysis or a transplant, sometimes called ESRD).

Medicare Advantage Plan (Part C)—A type of Medicare health plan offered by a private company that contracts with Medicare to provide you with all your Medicare Part A and Part B benefits. Medicare Advantage Plans include Health Maintenance Organizations, Preferred Provider Organizations, Private Fee-for-Service Plans, Special Needs Plans, and Medicare Medical Savings Account Plans. If you're enrolled in a Medicare Advantage Plan, most Medicare services are covered through the plan and aren't paid for under Original Medicare. Most Medicare Advantage Plans offer prescription drug coverage.

Medicare Cost Plan—A type of Medicare health plan available in some areas. In a Medicare Cost Plan, if you get services outside of the plan's network without a referral, your Medicare-covered services will be paid for under Original Medicare (your Cost Plan pays for emergency services or urgently-needed services).

Definitions

Medicare health plan—Generally, a plan offered by a private company that contracts with Medicare to provide Part A and Part B benefits to people with Medicare who enroll in the plan. Medicare health plans include all Medicare Advantage Plans, Medicare Cost Plans, and Demonstration/Pilot Programs. Programs of All-inclusive Care for the Elderly (PACE) organizations are special types of Medicare health plans that can be offered by public or private entities and provide Part D and other benefits in addition to Part A and Part B benefits.

Medicare Medical Savings Account (MSA) Plan—MSA Plans combine a high deductible Medicare Advantage Plan and a bank account. The plan deposits money from Medicare into the account. You can use the money in this account to pay for your health care costs, but only Medicare-covered expenses count toward your deductible. The amount deposited is usually less than your deductible amount so you generally will have to pay out-of-pocket before your coverage begins.

Medicare Part A (Hospital Insurance)—Part A covers inpatient hospital stays, care in a skilled nursing facility, hospice care, and some home health care.

Medicare Part B (Medical Insurance)—Part B covers certain doctors' services, outpatient care, medical supplies, and preventive services.

Medicare prescription drug coverage (Part D)—Optional benefits for prescription drugs available to all people with Medicare for an additional charge. This coverage is offered by insurance companies and other private companies approved by Medicare.

Medicare Prescription Drug Plan (Part D)—Part D adds prescription drug coverage to Original Medicare, some Medicare Cost Plans, some Medicare Private-Fee-for-Service Plans, and Medicare Medical Savings Account Plans. These plans are offered by insurance companies and other private companies approved by Medicare. Medicare Advantage Plans may also offer prescription drug coverage that follows the same rules as Medicare Prescription Drug Plans.

Medicare Private Fee-for-Service (PFFS) Plan—A type of Medicare Advantage Plan (Part C) in which you can generally go to any doctor or hospital you could go to if you had Original Medicare, if the doctor or hospital agrees to treat you. The plan determines how much it will pay doctors and hospitals, and how much you must pay when you get care. A Private Fee-For-Service Plan is very different than Original Medicare, and you must follow the plan rules carefully when you go for health care services. When you're in a Private Fee-For-Service Plan, you may pay more or less for Medicare-covered benefits than in Original Medicare.

Definitions

Medigap policy—Medicare Supplement Insurance sold by private insurance companies to fill "gaps" in Original Medicare coverage. Some Medigap policies sold before January 1, 2006, have prescription drug coverage. Policies sold on or after January 1, 2006, don't have prescription drug coverage.

Original Medicare—Original Medicare is a fee-for-service coverage under a fee-for-service health plan that has two parts: Part A (Hospital Insurance) and Part B (Medical Insurance). After you pay a deductible, Medicare pays its share of the Medicare-approved amount, and you pay your share (coinsurance and deductibles).

Penalty—An amount added to your monthly premium for Medicare Part B or a Medicare drug plan (Part D), if you don't join when you're first eligible. You pay this higher amount as long as you have Medicare. There are some exceptions.

Premium—The periodic payment to Medicare, an insurance company, or a health care plan for health or prescription drug coverage.

Programs of All-inclusive Care for the Elderly (PACE)—A special type of health plan that provides all the care and services covered by Medicare and Medicaid as well as additional medically necessary care and services based on your needs as determined by an interdisciplinary team. PACE serves frail older adults who need nursing home services but are capable of living in the community. PACE combines medical, social, and long-term care services and prescription drug coverage.

State Health Insurance Assistance Program (SHIP)—A state program that gets money from the Federal government to give free local health insurance counseling to people with Medicare.

State Medical Assistance (Medicaid) office—A state or local agency that can give information about, and assist with applications for, Medicaid programs that help pay medical bills for people with limited income and resources.

State Pharmaceutical Assistance Program (SPAP)—A state program that provides help paying for drug coverage based on financial need, age, or medical condition.

**U.S. DEPARTMENT OF
HEALTH AND HUMAN SERVICES**

Centers for Medicare & Medicaid Services
7500 Security Boulevard
Baltimore, Maryland 21244-1850

Official Business
Penalty for Private Use, $300

CMS Product No. 11109
Revised April 2016

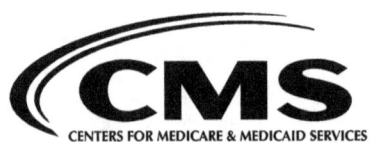

To get this booklet in Spanish, call 1-800-MEDICARE
(1-800-633-4227). TTY users should call 1-877-486-2048.

¿Necesita usted una copia de esta guía en Español?
Llame al 1-800-MEDICARE (1-800-633-4227). Los
usuarios de TTY deberán llamar al 1-877-486-2048.